COPING WITH EPILEPSY

Fiona Marshall is a freelance writer who has written widely on health, psychology and parenting. She is the author of seven books, four of them for Sheldon Press. She has written two other books on epilepsy, *Your Child: Epilepsy*, and *The Natural Way: Epilepsy*.

Overcoming Common Problems Series

For a full list of titles please contact
Sheldon Press, Marylebone Road, London NW1 4DU

Overcoming Common Problems

Coping with Epilepsy

Fiona Marshall
and
Dr Pamela Crawford

sheldon **PRESS**

Published in Great Britain in 2000 by
Sheldon Press,
Holy Trinity Church,
Marylebone Road, London NW1 4DU

Copyright © 2000 Fiona Marshall

British Library Cataloguing-in-Publication Data

A catalogue record for this book is available from the British Library

ISBN 0–85969–824–6

Typeset by Deltatype Limited, Birkenhead, Merseyside
Printed in Great Britain by
Biddles Ltd, Guildford and King's Lynn

Contents

To Michael

Introduction

A diagnosis of epilepsy can leave you and those around you reeling. Suddenly the boundaries of normality are changed, and everything you may previously have taken for granted is overturned, including health, identity, social expectations, relationships and career. How others perceive you, how you perceive yourself, whether you can now hope to achieve what you were aiming for – such fundamental concepts may be rocked to the core, and may leave you feeling very vulnerable.

The good news is that having epilepsy today is very different from having epilepsy in the past. Both medical treatment and the general public perception have changed dramatically over the past two or three decades. One area where this is especially relevant is drug treatment. In people with newly diagnosed epilepsy, up to 80 per cent become seizure-free on drugs, and there is now a broader range of drugs available for treatment. The last decade has seen the advent of seven new drugs, and many more novel compounds are also due to reach the marketplace. Many of the new drugs appear to have fewer side effects than existing and older ones, and, while of course the long-term side effects remain to be assessed, this does offer the prospect of effective and tolerable therapy for many. Surgery, though currently used for a minority, also offers hope for those with more resistant epilepsy, especially with the arrival of new surgical techniques.

Another important area of new and growing awareness is that of women with epilepsy. There is now much more acceptance of the fact that being a woman with epilepsy differs fundamentally from being a man with epilepsy. This book looks in some detail at issues affecting women, which in the past were by and large simply ignored.

Much more information exists on managing epilepsy yourself, especially in terms of how you can adjust your lifestyle so as to minimize the risk of seizures. There are also many excellent resources for people with epilepsy, including the national self-help groups listed at the back of this book. These groups have a very special and important role to play, offering support and up-to-date information which can help bridge any gaps between you and the doctor, and, perhaps most importantly, help you feel that you are not alone. Today, the social isolation that epilepsy used to threaten can be a thing of the past.

INTRODUCTION

Epilepsy does pose its own challenges, and this book aims to look at them in as constructive a way as possible. Much information about epilepsy exists, but is often lacking among many of those touched by the condition – in particular, not having information about your own type of epilepsy can be surprisingly common. There is still public ignorance about epilepsy, which sometimes has to be tackled vigorously for the person with epilepsy to be able to fulfil social activities and career prospects. Medical treatment may appear confusing and complex, and many people are daunted by the prospect of having to take drugs on a long-term basis.

But, one perception of epilepsy that has changed is that of 'epilepsy for life'. Many doctors used to believe that, once diagnosed, epilepsy was permanent. But newer work suggests that many people only have epilepsy for a limited period of their lives. An important UK study showed that in people who have been seizure-free for two or more years, at least 40 per cent were able successfully to stop therapy. In this study, people withdrew from drugs over at least a six-month period. (Withdrawal from anti-epileptic drugs should always be done slowly and under medical supervision to avoid withdrawal seizures.)

Obviously, the prognosis varies from individual to individual, but acceptance of your epilepsy does need to be balanced with hope. In practice, this may mean taking more responsibility for your condition, perhaps exploring lifestyle factors that seem to have an impact on your epilepsy, and this book contains practical information on strategies you might like to try, including diet and complementary therapies (which must indeed be complementary and not replace your current treatment – never give up your medication because you're trying an alternative remedy). It may also mean having your epilepsy re-evaluated by a neurologist who is a specialist in epilepsy – which can be another potential challenge. Again, this book suggests ways to get the most from your medical treatment, and how to create a true partnership with your medical carers.

Finally, perhaps one of epilepsy's greatest challenges is the boundaries it seems to impose. Again, this book aims to show that many boundaries are self-imposed, or due to over-protection from others – not caused by epilepsy. Research seems to agree that, in general, the more you know about epilepsy, the less likely you are to be intimidated by it. Learning about it can be vital to giving you a sense of control and freedom in life, and it is hoped that this book will go some way to helping you achieve this.

Acknowledgements

First, many thanks to my family for their support during the writing of this book. I would also like to acknowledge, with thanks, the help of the following: the British Epilepsy Association and the National Society for Epilepsy, especially Jo Lawrence-King of the NSE. I am indebted to *Women and Epilepsy* (Martin Dunitz) by Tim Betts, Consultant in Neuropsychiatry, and Clinical Director of Birmingham Brainwave, Birmingham University Seizure Clinic and Epilepsy Liaison Service, Queen Elizabeth Psychiatric Hospital, Birmingham, and Pam Crawford, Consultant Neurologist and Director of the Special Centre at York District Hospital Department of Neurology; also to work on women with epilepsy by Tim Betts, Dr Kate Smith, research fellow in epilepsy, and Cathy Fox, SRN, at Birmingham Brainwave. I would also like to acknowledge my debt to the detailed information and warm tone of books on epilepsy by, respectively, Anthony Hopkins and Richard Appleton, neurologist and paediatric neurologist; Dr John M. Freeman; and Brian Chappell and Dr Pamela Crawford (see Further reading). Thanks also to Julie Floyd, lecturer in horticulture at Harlow College, Middlesex. Above all, thanks to all the people who so generously shared their experiences of epilepsy, including Alan, Alison, Andrea, Audrey, Bronwen, Caroline, Catherine, Chris, Dawn, Damien, Diane, Elaine, Eveline, Fiona, George, Ivy, Kathryn, Jacky, Jan, Janice, John, Julie, Julia, Justine, Karolena, Linda, Lorraine, Vicky, Michael, Nicky, Pat, Paul, Sam, Sarah, Thomas, Valerie and William.

Fiona Marshall

1

Understanding epilepsy

The most common brain disorder in the world is the most misunderstood and neglected. Epilepsy is far more widespread than is generally realized, affecting 40 to 50 million people worldwide – around 1 in 200 of us. We probably all know someone with epilepsy, even though we may not be aware that they have the condition. Yet, myth and misunderstanding abound, sometimes even among the medical profession – even the best neurologists do not always understand epilepsy! Epilepsy can strike anyone at any time, but it is not an illness. It affects the brain, but it is not a mental or psychiatric disorder. It may sometimes be passed on from generation to generation, but it is not contagious. It is not usually curable, but in up to 80 per cent of cases it can be controlled effectively by drugs.

So what is epilepsy? Broadly, epilepsy means no more than a tendency to have seizures. This liability to seizures may be caused by many underlying brain dysfunctions. Epilepsy is a group of disorders, not a single condition. It covers a multitude of conditions to do with brain malfunction – in fact, asking what is epilepsy is rather like asking what is weather, when every day is different. It affects each person differently, with a wide range of symptoms and very varying degrees of severity. Epilepsy is best understood on an individual basis.

This is all the more so as epilepsy is a condition which affects not just many aspects of health, but also lifestyle issues such as relationships, education, careers and hobbies. In children and teenagers, for example, proper treatment of epilepsy is essential to allow them to fulfil their educational potential, learn how to form relationships, create confidence, and generally live life to the full.

For women, epilepsy has very particular implications in terms of sexual development, the menstrual cycle, contraception, fertility, pregnancy and the menopause. Until recently, the treatment of women with epilepsy tended to be the same as the treatment of men with epilepsy, despite the fact that 50 per cent of people with epilepsy are female. In practice, this meant that women were treated as if they were men, and their specific medical needs tended to be ignored or overlooked. However, there is now increasing recognition of the fact that having epilepsy is not the same for a woman as for a man, and treatment reflects this more, one of the most important areas being pre-conception counselling.

In older people, epilepsy has added relevance in that it may be a symptom of an underlying condition such as stroke. Early treatment may also help prevent physical damage from seizures, which may pose an additional danger to older people whose bones tend to be more brittle. Seizure control is also vital in terms of giving confidence to older people, who may risk isolation through fear of having a seizure or not being able to drive. This applies potentially to all with epilepsy but may have special relevance for older people.

Understanding epilepsy means different things to the affected person, and to the doctor. As with all medical conditions, the person affected views it from the inside, the doctor from the outside, although epilepsy may be singular in that the affected person often has no direct experience of what a seizure is like. If you lose consciousness during a seizure, you miss the essential symptom of your condition. This limited perception is often further clouded by lack of information about the condition, which can be surprisingly common even among people affected by it.

For people with epilepsy, epilepsy tends to be understood best in terms of its immediate impact. This may vary but potentially includes poor health, vulnerability, the constant dread of seizures, having to take daily medication, perhaps not being able to drive, being uncertain about a career, lacking confidence in relationships. This sounds a daunting list. But, it must be emphasized that it by no means applies to everyone with epilepsy. Self-imposed limitations (along with over-protection from others) may do more to affect a person's experience of epilepsy than almost any other factor. This means that how the individual approaches his or her epilepsy can be key both in understanding and managing it, and it is hoped that this book will provide some tools with which to tackle these aims in a positive and effective way.

What happens in epilepsy

Epilepsy is when the brain, which works by electricity, produces sudden bursts of electrical energy or 'storms' which disrupt its normal workings. Epilepsy is usually viewed as a symptom of underlying neurological damage or disorder, not a disease in its own right, although in some cases the cause can be an illness with a genetic component. The brain itself is a highly complex and sensitive organ which controls and regulates all our movements and sensations, as well

2

as unconscious body functions such as heartbeat and breathing. It is the seat of memory, thoughts and emotions, and its smooth working, which most of us take for granted, is absolutely fundamental to our sense of our own identity, or 'I am'. When all this is thrown into chaos, as it is when a seizure strikes, small wonder that a person may feel totally disorientated, as all the mechanics and signals normally used to recognize the world are obliterated.

Normally, the brain works by a constant exchange of electric signals between its different components – an ongoing 'chatter' between the millions of neurons or brain cells. This 'chatter' is in the form of neurotransmitters, chemicals which send or stop messages. The right balance between different types of neurotransmitters is normally what keeps the whole 'conversation' going. But, sometimes, the balance is disrupted by a sudden abnormal electrical discharge or 'storm' from a group of cells, and the result is a seizure. Depending on which part of the brain is affected, and how, the person may experience changes in bodily function and consciousness, sometimes severe, sometimes more mild.

About the brain

There are three parts of the brain – the cerebrum, the cerebellum and the brainstem, with the cerebrum being more likely to be affected by seizure activity.

- *The cerebrum* is the main mass of the brain and so is the major part governing how we behave and think. It contains the two hemispheres, joined together at the base by the thick, multi-fibred corpus callosum. Each hemisphere is divided into four lobes which govern particular functions. The frontal lobes control voluntary movements, and some aspects of personality and emotions. The parietal lobes are involved in body sensations such as feeling and touch as well as in fine manual skills such as writing. The temporal lobes have to do with memory, understanding, speech, emotions, sexual feelings, taste and smell. The occipital lobes are responsible for sight – both what is seen, and how sights are interpreted. Some forms of epilepsy, where partial seizures are involved (see Chapter 2 for a description of seizure types), may start from any one of these lobes, so bringing about disturbances in sensation.

- *The cerebellum*, just beneath the two hemispheres, has to do with the control of movements. Its main function is to co-ordinate the many muscular actions needed to make any movement from lifting a fork to doing the high jump. It is also concerned with balance. The cerebellum operates at an unconscious level and processes a great deal of information from several different sources, such as the eyes, the ears, all the muscles, and different parts of the cerebrum. Disturbance of the cerebellum causes ataxia, or a loss of co-ordination which can involve clumsiness, staggering or severe tremor.

- *The brainstem* is the oldest part of the brain and connects the cerebrum and cerebellum with the spinal cord. It controls basic functions such as breathing and heartbeat and also co-ordinates other activities such as eye and tongue movements. Damage to this part of the brain is always serious.

Why epilepsy develops

It is natural to ask 'Why?' when epilepsy strikes. There is a need to make sense of a condition which has descended without apparent rhyme or reason, and so most people will search for cause and effect when it comes to their epilepsy. We also tend to expect that modern medicine has an answer for everything. But, it is not always possible to find a convincing cause – in fact, a known cause for epilepsy can be discovered only in 25–30 per cent of cases, and even then it may often be more accurate to call it a precipitating factor. For example, not everyone who receives a blow to the head will suffer epilepsy as a result. But, a severe blow to an individual who has a predetermined susceptibility to epilepsy may result in epilepsy. Or, the development of epilepsy may in fact be coincidental, but, because the person has had a blow to the head a few weeks before, he or she will automatically assume that this blow is the cause. This need to find a cause which makes it all more understandable can sometimes be a cause of disagreement between patient and doctor.

Daphne was convinced that her epilepsy began after a course of antibiotics but every doctor she met told her it was just coincidence. So who was right? Do you trust the intuition of Daphne or the experience of the doctors? In the end, Daphne saw a different neurologist when she moved who told her that seizures could in fact result from high doses of penicillin, though normally they should stop once the offending drug had been withdrawn. In this case, her neurologist concluded that the penicillin might well have been the causative factor in precipitating epilepsy, but that she must have a naturally low seizure threshold.

'Seizure threshold', sometimes known as 'convulsive threshold', is the brain's individual level of sensitivity to seizures, and is a major factor in the development of epilepsy. Seizure threshold is genetically determined. However, everyone is capable of having an epileptic seizure in certain conditions, for example in a high fever, or after heavy prolonged drinking. But, some people's seizure threshold is lower than others, in which case those people may be more predisposed to having seizures.

People with epilepsy have a lower than normal seizure threshold, so making the brain cells more likely to 'fire' at a lower level of stimulus. Various factors affect seizure threshold, including age – the younger the person, the lower the threshold may be, making a seizure more likely, which may help explain why epilepsy starting in childhood is often outgrown as the brain matures. Other factors include brain scarring and genetic inheritance.

Genetic causes of epilepsy is an area of growing importance. Various genes have been identified as being linked with certain forms of epilepsy: benign neonatal familial convulsions, which affect newborns but disappear by three months, and progressive myoclonus epilepsy, both rare forms of epilepsy. Juvenile myoclonic epilepsy (JME) is also known to have a genetic base, as is primary generalized epilepsy. Some brain disease may also be inherited, such as tuberous sclerosis. On the whole, though, people are more likely to inherit a genetic predisposition to epilepsy than epilepsy itself. Having epilepsy in the family means there is a slight chance it might be passed on, but it is by no means certain. For example, of two identical twins, one might have epilepsy and the other not.

Research is constantly adding to understanding of the mechanics of epilepsy, and it is now believed that very subtle malformations in brain development in the baby before birth are often the underlying cause of epilepsy. One such cause is neuronal migration, when pockets of brain cells which should go to one destination end up in another, so that they are in the wrong location or with wrong connections. These are often tiny, too subtle to be picked up even by modern scanning methods. Nevertheless they result in seizures.

In a few cases, it's also thought that what happens in pregnancy may affect the baby, including the mother having viral or bacterial infections during pregnancy, drinking too much, or using illegal drugs. However, this is where the need to find a cause can play havoc with the emotions – for example, many women automatically blame themselves for their child's epilepsy, or spend their pregnancy worrying needlessly about some minor incident (such as a few drinks in early pregnancy) which they fear will have damaged the baby. It must be emphasized that in most cases, the foetus is very hardy, and unlikely to be damaged by the mother's behaviour.

What about known causes? Depending on what kind of seizure threshold you may have inherited, some environmental trigger or damage is often needed for seizures to start. This kind of damage varies according to age and circumstances. One of the most common causes of epilepsy in adults is head trauma owing to accidents such as car accidents or falls. Not every random blow will result in epilepsy – it has to be severe enough to cause scarring of the brain tissue. Stroke, which interrupts blood flow to the brain, is the most common cause of epilepsy in older people. Other causes include brain tumour, over-exposure to toxins such as lead or aluminium, alcohol poisoning or repeated heavy drinking; or 'recreational' drugs such as Ecstasy or cocaine. It is very unlikely that emotional trauma, such as rape, may trigger epilepsy but it can precipitate seizures in someone with epilepsy. (This kind of shock may also trigger a different kind of seizure which is psychological in nature, not epileptic – see Chapter 3, which looks at epileptic and non-epileptic seizures.) In babies and young children, common causes include birth trauma involving lack of oxygen (anoxia), congenital central nervous system malformations, and abnormalities in the metabolism – blood chemical abnormalities such as low calcium, magnesium or glucose, which may alter the balance of the blood or its chemical structure. Seizures may also result from infections which may damage the nerve cells in the brain, such as meningitis, viral encephalitis, lupus erythematosus and less frequently mumps, measles, diphtheria and others.

Such events may leave a scar or lesion on the brain which becomes an 'epileptic focus' – an identifiable point from which seizures may start. When doctors can identify the underlying disorder, the condition is referred to as symptomatic epilepsy, in contrast to idiopathic epilepsy, which simply means epilepsy of unknown cause, and cryptogenic epilepsy, when a cause is suspected but none can be found.

Some causes are transient, for example, a high fever or head trauma, and the resulting seizures are sometimes called 'provoked seizures'. This means that when what causes the seizure goes, you will get better.

Generally, it may often be better not to be able to find a cause. Seizures of unknown cause – more than 70 per cent of all seizures – are most likely to remit (stop spontaneously) and most likely to be easily controlled by one drug; and the causes which can be found are often worse than the ones which can't, as they may indicate a neurological problem such as stroke, infection, tumour or blood vessel problem.

Links with other conditions

Because epilepsy is sometimes related to underlying brain damage or disorder, it may sometimes accompany other problems also caused by brain malfunction, such as learning disability. About 30 per cent of people with a learning disability have epilepsy, and, in those with a severe learning disability, the number of those with epilepsy rises to 80 per cent. Generally, epilepsy is far more common, and frequently more severe, in people who have other conditions which affect the brain, such a cerebral palsy and cerebrovascular disease (stroke) – though these conditions co-exist, and do not actually cause each other. But anyone can develop epilepsy, whatever their level of intelligence.

Epilepsy is sometimes linked to other conditions, too. For example, there is a higher incidence of epilepsy in children with autism, especially around adolescence, and some researchers believe that autism is due to an abnormality in the brain itself, or a disturbance in the body chemistry which affects the brain. Recently, researchers have focused on the brain structure of people with autism. Using modern brain-scanning techniques, researchers have found that there may be a structural difference in the cerebellum, though findings are not specific enough for scans to diagnose autism. However, neurological damage is now believed to be the cause of autism, just as with epilepsy.

Another link is with migraine – in fact, neurologist Oliver Sacks describes migraine as 'epilepsy in slow motion', as there are some similarities in brainwave patterns. A number of older studies have found that migraine sufferers had a higher prevalence of epilepsy, though these studies have been criticized as flawed. Like epilepsy, migraine may start with an aura or warning such as visual disturbance, although in migraine consciousness is hardly ever lost, as it often is in an epileptic seizure. There has also been speculation that there may be a common genetic component for epilepsy and migraine. However, a recent American study of nearly 2,000 people found that the risk of epilepsy in relatives was not associated with a history of migraine, with the exception of the sons of female migraineurs, people do not share a genetic susceptibility to both migraine and epilepsy, so leaving unclear the links between migraine and epilepsy. All this said, it is by no means uncommon for people with epilepsy to experience migraine and/or severe headaches, either as part of a seizure or alone.

Who has epilepsy?

Although epilepsy can start at any point during a person's life, most epilepsy is diagnosed in childhood, and most of all in the first year of life – around 140 out of every 100,000 babies under the age of one are diagnosed with epilepsy per year. This drops to 40 adults per 100,000. However, recent reports have shown that epilepsy is increasing in older people, who account for a quarter of all new diagnoses, according to a survey by the National Society for Epilepsy. The condition is twice as common in older people than it is in the population as a whole.

It may be even more common than is documented, because some of it probably goes unrecognized. Diagnosing epilepsy in the elderly can be difficult. In many cases the seizures are mild, and, while this is excellent news in terms of control, it may also mean that it's not so easy to spot them for what they are. Aunt Alice's daydreaming, Gran's 'funny turns', may form part of family folklore and certainly not be seen to warrant medical investigation. We tend to expect illness and absent-mindedness in older people as a matter of course. However, epilepsy in later life may well be among the more preventable cases of the condition. The older we get, the more liable we become to decreased fitness and health, but, in particular, epilepsy in the older person is often due to cerebrovascular disease which leads to small scars in the brain. In general, the risk of epilepsy in older people may be reduced with proper attention to lifestyle, including healthy eating, enough exercise, not smoking, and drinking alcohol moderately. Paying attention to lifestyle issues may help people of any age gain better seizure control and improve general health, and may also prevent your epilepsy getting worse in older age. There's more on healthy lifestyle in Chapter 7.

Epilepsy is divided almost equally betwen the sexes, though a few epilepsy syndromes occur exclusively in girls. Epilepsy is slightly more common in men, and there are various reasons why this may be so. One reason is that men are more likely to suffer head injury and brain infection. Another theory is that the brains of boy and girl babies

8

develop differently in the womb due to differences in male and female sex hormones. The brain matures more rapidly in girl babies than boy ones, so that girls are less vulnerable to perinatal anoxia (lack of oxygen around birth) which can damage developing areas of the brain. The Y chromosome which produces maleness in unborn babies also slows development down, so that boys are born around two to three weeks behind in maturity than girls, so making them more vulnerable to injury. This vulnerability persists into adulthood – one study showed that, in women, 50 per cent of the risk of developing epilepsy was past by the time they were 19, but in men, this did not happen until they were 24. This risk is thought to outweigh men's larger brain size. Another study showed that the brains of men and women only become the same size when they are 100, when they have both shrunk enough to be similar! There is some evidence that the prognosis or outlook is slightly worse in women, and it has been suggested that this is because women's brains are tougher, a more severe event is needed to precipitate the epilepsy. But, in practice, most of these differences are slight – again, each person with epilepsy represents an individual case, and should be treated as such.

Despite its high prevalence, epilepsy, traditionally the 'Cinderella' of the health service, attracts little by way of research money – out of the UK's annual £2 billion medical research budget only £336,000 is spent on epilepsy, less than £1 per person with epilepsy, and comparing unfavourably with say the £250 per person with muscular dystrophy and £140 per person with multiple sclerosis.

A recent survey of health managers in the UK revealed that only 5 per cent had set service standards for epilepsy. However, this may change as epilepsy achieves greater media coverage and public interest, something which is taking place – over the past few years, according to the National Society for Epilepsy, epilepsy has become an 'interesting' subject as genetic research and modern brain-scanning methods reveal more about the condition.

Can epilepsy be fatal?

The vast majority of people with epilepsy will have no need to consider this question, but it is worth discussing in view of SUDEP (Sudden Unexplained Death in Epilepsy) which in recent years has received quite a lot of publicity, and has, not unnaturally, alarmed many people.

SUDEP is a rare phenomenon whereby people with epilepsy, usually young and in relatively good health, die without warning, quite often when asleep at night and unwitnessed. It is not to be confused with Sudden Death Syndrome, which like SUDEP often affects young people, but is thought to be due to previously hidden cardiac trouble. SUDEP was known about in 1868, a time when epilepsy was viewed almost as being on a par with leprosy and many with epilepsy were kept in colonies away from the community. So, although the subject received scientific attention, stigma meant that death associated with epilepsy was kept under wraps and forgotten about as much as possible. The twentieth century brought the increasing medicalization of epilepsy, new anti-epileptic drugs, and a move by those concerned with epilepsy to present it in a positive, upbeat light in order to fight ignorance and stigma in the general community. The risks of mortality were played down, but some feel it is now time that the balance is redressed.

There seem to be two basic attitudes to SUDEP among both medical professionals and people affected by epilepsy. The first is that you have about as much chance of dying of SUDEP as being run over by a bus, and that is not worth spending your life worrying about it. Many people with epilepsy suffer enough from over-protection by families, partners and friends, and the last thing they need is the additional burden of anxiety about suddenly dying. The second view – more prevalent among those who have actually had their lives touched by SUDEP – is that ignorance about and indifference to SUDEP merely reflects the neglect of epilepsy in general, and that lack of research only serves to hide the true figures of SUDEP and to keep going the status quo of silence and misinformation around these deaths. People who have lost a loved one to SUDEP have been traumatized as much by the lack of information and support as by anything else, and even the cause of death is often not acknowledged, as deaths from SUDEP are still often attributed to other causes such as asphyxia (suffocation) on death certificates.

Both views exist in the face of overwhelming lack of information. While the chances of anyone dying 'from epilepsy' are extremely few and far between, many neurologists and people with epilepsy feel there is a great need for further education and openness if SUDEP is to be tackled, and, if possible, prevented. In addition, litigation is becoming an issue, especially in the US, where cases have focused on the risks of withdrawal of medication and doctors' failure to give information about the possible risks of SUDEP. Doctors in the UK are currently calling for a confidential enquiry into SUDEP to help establish its causes. There is no doubt that this would throw into focus the general lack of medical resources for epilepsy in the UK, which has only 12 epilepsy clinics compared with, for example, 114 for diabetes. One issue which an inquiry might address is the possibility of sub-optimal medical care, such as patients being on the wrong drugs or the wrong dose. The majority of patients are seen by hospital doctors who have no specialist training in epilepsy. Another issue is long waiting lists for appointments with neurologists – some people have died while waiting for their first appointment, which has obvious implications for how suspected or newly diagnosed epilepsy should be handled. One of the main questions is how preventable the deaths are, and which preventative measures could be taken, from a night monitor to assess seizure activity and respiration, to ensuring someone is with the person after a seizure, to new drugs or general resources for epilepsy care. Findings might have major implications for some people with epilepsy, such as how safe it would be to live alone, or whether some individuals might need special links with emergency care.

However, this is all speculative until the causes of SUDEP can be established more precisely. SUDEP is thought to take place during or immediately after a seizure. Research so far suggests that cardiac arrhythmias (changes in heart rate) are the most likely cause, possibly caused or made worse by disorganized electrical brain activity during a seizure – certain nerve connections from parts of the brain affect blood flow and heart activity. Another possible cause is that hormones released during a seizure affect heart rhythm and that this, combined with the fact that a seizure causes breathing to pause, may sometimes be enough to cause death.

SUDEP is particularly distressing as it goes against all traditional wisdom about seizures not being life-threatening. It must be emphasized that it is very rare for someone to die during a seizure, though people who have lost a loved one to SUDEP will have a different perception of this – it happened to them. How common is SUDEP? It is difficult to establish this because of lack of research and because of the fact that the deaths are often not recognized as being from SUDEP. In 1996, the known figures were 969 deaths in the UK (twice those of cot death and the same as the combined mortality figures for cot deaths and HIV). The estimated risk is varying, from 1 in 1,000 for all people with epilepsy, to 1 in 200 for those at highest risk. However, a study at the Mayo Clinic, Rochester, USA found that SUDEP was a rare cause of death among people with epilepsy, accounting for just 1.7 per cent of deaths, but that exceeds the expected rate of sudden death in the general population by nearly 24 times.

SUDEP also needs to be seen in context along with general mortality risks of epilepsy. People with epilepsy do have a greater statistical risk of premature death, usually said to be two to four times greater than that of the average population. Some of this is attributable to accidents during seizures, such as drowning or road accidents. Some mortality risk also relates to how well epilepsy is controlled, as people with uncontrolled chronic epilepsy are an estimated eight times more likely to die than their peers. Status epilepticus, a form of prolonged seizure, is also associated with a greater risk of death. However, all these figures tend to relate more to those with very severe epilepsy or to those whose epilepsy involves underlying central nervous system disease such as brain tumours or stroke. Those with well-controlled epilepsy, around 80 per cent of those with epilepsy, have normal life expectancy.

What is known about SUDEP does suggest that certain people are more likely to be at risk: men aged 20–40; people with poorly controlled tonic-clonic seizures; those with a history of alcoholism; people who do not take medication regularly; and those whose epilepsy is caused by a structural disorder in the brain. Until more is known about SUDEP, general preventative advice is usually given as follows:

- get seizures under control as far as possible;
- take medication regularly;
- avoid sudden drug withdrawal.

Does epilepsy ever get better?

Caroline used to have tonic-clonic seizures which seemed to be made worse by her anticonvulsant drugs, phenytoin and carbamazepine. Her seizures stopped when she withdrew from her medication and paid real, detailed attention to her diet, including specially prescribed supplements under the guidance of a nutritionist. She now only has seizures when exposed to two particular triggers, the smell of wet paint and cough medicine, but, for her, epilepsy is generally a thing of the past.

Epilepsy is like a marriage – only there's no question of divorce. Epilepsy won't pack its bags and walk out on you. It's definitely here to say, for life, for better or worse. For me, it's a question of, have a seizure, then pick myself up and get on with my daily activities on the farm as if nothing had happened – several times a day.
Bronwen

What is so daunting about a diagnosis of epilepsy is that it implies a disorder which will last for life. But, this is another of the areas where thinking about epilepsy has changed in recent years. Many doctors feel that 'epilepsy for life' reflects undue pessimism, stemming from older research which focused on people with the worst kind of epilepsy, usually institutionalized and treated with older drugs. It is now known that epilepsy often gets better, that many people do not need to take medication all their lives, and that many people who developed epilepsy in childhood do outgrow it. Around 70 per cent of children who have a first seizure never have another, while many people have only a handful of seizures in their lives.

Major studies of the population in general have shown that the vast majority of people do have an excellent chance of achieving a long period of seizure freedom. According to one long-term study in Olmstead county, USA, several findings pointed to the possibility of remission or a period of seizure freedom. According to this study:

- one year after diagnosis, 42 per cent of people entered a seizure-free period which lasted for at least five years;
- the probability of being seizure-free was 61 per cent at 10 years and 70 per cent 20 years after diagnosis;
- 20 years after diagnosis 50 per cent of people had been seizure-free without medication for at least five years.

Other studies on remission have shown that 92 per cent of all those who had seizures had achieved remission lasting at least one year, while nearly 70 per cent enjoyed a four-year remission.

If your epilepsy is not currently controlled, or you feel your prognosis is not good, these figures may seem very frustrating. However, scientists are constantly researching new drugs and surgical methods aimed at intractable epilepsy, and it is always possible that a really competent re-evaluation of your epilepsy by a specialist may lead to some of the newer treatments being more effective.

The prognosis may depend on various factors. One is the underlying cause of the epilepsy. For example, if this is due to an underlying illness, then treating this successfully will cure the epilepsy. Again, some types of epilepsy may mean that a person is a candidate for surgery, which can sometimes effectively cure the epilepsy. Generally, while doctors cannot predict who will continue to have seizures and who will not, they usually feel that the sooner epilepsy is diagnosed, the better it can be controlled. Starting treatment sooner rather than later is often thought to make for a better prognosis and more likely remission – though not all doctors agree. Some believe that treatment should be delayed, and there's more on this complex question in Chapter 3, which deals with treatment.

Some types of epilepsy carry a better remission rate than others. For example, two kinds of epilepsy which largely affect children – absence seizures and Benign Rolandic Epilepsy of Childhood (BREC) – are outgrown by 75–100 per cent of all those affected by the teenage years. Other factors which indicate a good prognosis include:

- having epilepsy which starts after 5 years of age but before 13;
- seizure types involving absence or tonic-clonic seizures (see Chapter 2 for definition of seizures);
- having seizures which are easily controlled by one drug;
- a family history of epilepsy;
- not having any known cause for epilepsy;
- having a normal or near-normal EEG;
- not having any evidence of neurological problems.

Anecdotal evidence suggests that remission can sometimes be an individual affair, maybe depending on psychological as well as physiological factors. Some people, like Caroline mentioned above, have managed to put epilepsy behind them by changing aspects of their lifestyle. While this may not 'cure' epilepsy in everyone, tackling general health and lifestyle issues can certainly help. There is a great deal you can do to take control of your own wellbeing and so help improve epilepsy, and this book suggests many ways you can do this.

2

Seizures

The seizures start with a feeling of time slowing down immensely while everything becomes very familiar and I know that everything is happening in slow motion as it has done many times before – what they call *déjà vu*. I then get a feeling of warmth and tightness in the pit of my stomach and then a sudden feeling of terror. I know 'it's' going to happen again and I start to panic and feel I can't breathe.
Julie

I have a short warning. Everything is amplified tremendously and then the visions start, with a view of a city in ruins. I can never remember afterwards exactly what I see after that. When I come round I'm often extremely disorientated, forget my name and suffer extreme emotional confusion and usually tears.
Anthea

It's like people whispering, that's the nearest I can get to it. There's a kind of great hush, then it's like people going 'fwish fwish fwish' in my ears for about 30 seconds before I black out. After a seizure I feel disorientated, sounds are muffled, and I have a headache. I have little memory of the actual seizure, but as I am semi-conscious when I recover, I can realize that something is wrong and ask others to verify it.
Lorraine

My chest and stomach start tightening. I feel a kind of exultation, and an intense feeling of love and radiance.
Alan

People sound as if they're talking through water or through some other medium – I know people are speaking to me but the words are distorted. Then I start to feel sick and giddy, and that I'm losing it. Sometimes I have enough time to tell those around me that I'm going.
William

I get a foul smell, like rotting eggs, followed by a rising or surging sensation in my stomach, a bit like being on a rollercoaster. Then I feel as if I'm being sucked into a narrowing tunnel. When I come round, my memory for the hour before the seizure is extremely hazy.
Audrey

I suffer confusion and automatic behaviour following a seizure – I have had several accusations, some in writing, of being drunk on duty.
Janice

Not everyone can describe their seizure experience. The above quotations all come from people whose epilepsy affects a part of their brain either before or during a seizure – not enough for them to lose consciousness entirely, but enough for their consciousness to be disturbed in all kinds of unusual ways. A seizure can affect any part of the brain, and the variety of experiences described above reflect that – what the person feels depends on which part of the brain is being affected by the seizure. Hence, smelling bad smells is because the olfactory or smell area of the brain is being irritated by the seizure activity, while hallucinations may be because of seizure activity in the memory area.

But, the above quotations don't apply to all seizures. There are several different types of seizure, many of which may happen without any warning. The first the person may know of the seizure is coming round, perhaps in utter confusion and with a pounding headache, with a group of frightened people around. Or the person may just pause in his or her everyday activities for a few seconds, not even realizing that he or she is having a seizure. Neither may others. Seizures can go unrecognized for years, masquerading as mildly annoying personal habits such as daydreaming, fidgeting, and not listening or replying to what is said. Or, seizures can be so dramatic, with noise, convulsions and a blue face, that witnesses are convinced the person is dying.

Seizures are bursts of excessive, chaotic, electrical energy which interrupt normal brain activity, and are the main sign that epilepsy is present. Because they can affect any part of the brain, or all of it, seizures can cause disruptions to personality, mood, memory, sensations or movement – all that is fundamental to the freedom of being which most people take for granted. In addition, the person with epilepsy may suffer accompanying symptoms before or after the attack. These vary enormously – seeing or hearing what is not there, smelling

16

odd, sickening smells, feeling giddy or sick, feeling depersonalized or 'spaced out', suffering headaches or exhaustion. A person may have just one type of seizure, or several types. Anyone can have a seizure under certain conditions (such as too much alcohol) and 1 in 20 people have a seizure at some point during their lives, though they may never have another and may not be diagnosed with epilepsy. Of those who are diagnosed, around 75 per cent have their first seizure by the age of 20.

While there are at least 40 different classifiable seizure types, they tend to be divided into two main kinds depending on how much of the brain they affect: *generalized*, when the whole of the brain is involved and consciousness is disturbed or lost; and *partial*, when part of the brain is involved and consciousness may or may not be disturbed. These two main categories subdivide into other different types of seizure, as the next section explains.

Types of seizures

A specific classification system of the different seizures has been adopted by the International League Against Epilepsy (ILAE), an organization for health professionals concerned with epilepsy. The International Classification of Epileptic Seizures has been widely used by the medical community since its introduction in 1981, as has the International Classification of Epilepsies, Epileptic Syndromes, and Related Disorders which was adopted in 1989. Since then, however, advances in diagnostic technology, and recent research into neuronal mechanisms of epilepsy and genetics have meant that this classification is being refined and revised. Most recently, too, genetic discoveries may mean that some types of epilepsy can be reclassified as diseases which may be inherited, though these are generally in a minority.

For practical purposes, though, the basic structure of the existing classification is unlikely to change, and is described as follows.

Generalized seizures

There are six major types of generalized seizures, which, because they affect the entire brain, often result in the person falling down. 'The fall' was for centuries noted as essential to a diagnosis of epilepsy, and a tonic-clonic seizure, in which the fall is unmistakeable, is still what many people think of as epilepsy today.

- *Absence seizures* involve a brief loss of awareness for a few seconds, though they may last perhaps up to 20 seconds. They typically happen dozens or even hundreds of times a day. They may be accompanied by little involuntary movements such as blinking, chewing movements, or turning of the head. These seizures may happen so quickly that the person, and sometimes others around him, may not notice that anything has happened. On the other hand, this is the type of seizure which is most commonly mistaken for daydreaming or inattentiveness. Someone having this kind of seizure is completely unaware of people and things around him, but quickly returns to full consciousness after the attack. They usually start in childhood.

- *Myoclonic seizures* involve sudden jerky movements of any muscles in the body ('myo' means muscle and 'clonic' means convulsive or jerking), though they usually affect the arms or legs, and sometimes the head. For example, the person may suddenly fling up both arms, or nod his head. The seizures are fleeting, lasting up to one second. Myoclonic attacks may happen on their own or with other generalized seizures such as absence seizures. If consciousness is lost, it is only for a few seconds. The person recovers immediately, and the seizure is not usually followed by drowsiness or sleepiness. These seizures may occur many times a day.

- *Atonic or astatic or akinetic seizures* involve a sudden brief loss of muscle control, causing the person to fall suddenly to the ground – the word 'atonic' literally means lack of muscle tone. Because they cause such sudden, abrupt falls, these seizures are also called drop attacks. The seizures last a few seconds, but the sudden drop can cause cuts and bruises to the head and face. Because atonic seizures are hard to control and may occur many times during the day, some children and adults with this type of seizure wear helmets to protect their faces and foreheads.

- *Tonic seizures* involve a sudden stiffening of the limbs or whole body, again causing a fall. This seizure usually lasts for 5–10 seconds.

- *Clonic seizures* are when the muscles contract repeatedly and rhythmically so that the legs and arms, or sometimes the whole body, jerks or twitches. These usually last from 30 seconds to 2 minutes, occasionally longer.

18

- **Tonic-clonic seizures** (*'grand mal'*) involve a sudden overall contracting ('tonic' means contracting) of all the person's muscles, which means the person falls to the ground. Because the muscles around the lungs tighten, the air is forced out, causing an involuntary cry (the *'cri épileptique'* or epileptic cry like 'the fall' was for centuries noted as an essential component of an epileptic seizure) – the teeth clench as the jaw muscles contract, and breathing stops momentarily, making the person turn blue (cyanosis). Sweating, dribbling saliva may happen, or bladder or bowel control may be lost. All this forms the 'tonic' (contracting) part of the seizure, which lasts a couple of minutes and then passes into the 'clonic' (convulsive) phase, when the leg, arm and trunk muscles convulse rhythmically. The person may then lie unconscious, breathing hard as colour and consciousness gradually return. Confusion, exhaustion, irritability, painful muscles or headache are quite common after the seizure, which normally lasts 1–3 minutes.

Partial (focal) seizures

Partial seizures as the name implies start from a part of the brain, though they may also spread throughout the whole brain, becoming a *secondary generalized* seizure. Partial seizures may involve changes in awareness, movement or feeling, and, depending on whether awareness is affected, may be further subdivided into *simple* and *complex*.

- **Simple partial seizures** affect a small area of the brain, starting from one of the four lobes in one hemisphere but do not affect a person's consciousness or awareness. Although unable to control movements or to stop the seizure, the person remains conscious and may even be able to describe to someone else what is going on. Most simple partial seizures involve unusual sensations – the size or shape of things may look distorted, or the person may 'see' people or things that are not there. He may hear strange sounds or have a feeling that what is happening around him has somehow happened before (*déjà vu*). On the other hand, familiar surroundings may suddenly seem unfamiliar (*jamais vu*). He or she may feel an odd sensation in the stomach or on the skin. A simple partial seizure can also affect feelings, for example causing fear, dread, a sense of impending doom, anger, or, on the other hand, joy or elation. These seizures are also sometimes called *simple partial sensory seizures*, and may also

19

form the *aura*, or warning, of a further seizure, which happens if the seizure activity spreads over both halves of the brain (hemispheres) so that the person loses consciousness, when the seizure is known as a *secondary generalized seizure*. A simple partial seizure may also spread and become a complex partial seizure (see below).

The reason for the sometimes frightening sensations involved in simple partial seizures (or auras) is that unusual electrical activity is taking place in parts of the brain that control seeing, hearing, memory or sensation. The quotes at the start of this chapter describe auras and simple partial seizures, and show how a person's experience of this kind of seizure depends on which part of the brain is affected – specifically, which of the four lobes making up a hemisphere. Seizures which start in the *parietal lobe* may produce brief tingling in the arms or legs, or pins and needles down one side of the body, while if the *occipital lobe* is involved, visual disturbances may result such as seeing flashing lights. *Frontal lobe* seizures may involve body movements such as sudden thrashing of the body, bicycling movements of the legs, sudden stiff extension of an arm, or even crying out and running.

Temporal lobe seizures are the most common kind and involve most of the intense and complex changes of consciousness, including fear, panic, *déjà vu*, hallucinations and intensification of everyday experiences. The often visionary nature of these experiences has led to some interest in the creative or spiritual side of temporal lobe epilepsy (TLE), and some of the literature (see Further reading) looks at how these experiences have been expressed in poetry and painting by many people, some of them famous – Dostoevsky and van Gogh are the classic examples.

- **Complex partial seizures** do affect a person's consciousness or awareness. Sometimes a simple partial seizure may spread quickly to the areas which affect consciousness and develop into a complex partial seizure; sometimes, complex partial seizures will happen without any warning or aura.

  A complex partial seizure is one in which the electrical disturbance has spread far enough over the brain so that the person is unaware of events while the seizure is happening. They typically appear to be in a kind of trance or daze, or go through a series of movements over which they have no control, such as staring, chewing, pulling at clothing or walking around, looking confused or dazed; sometimes a person may mistakenly be thought drunk. Although the seizure lasts for only a minute or two, full awareness of the surroundings may not return for some time afterwards.

After a seizure

'Automatisms' (or 'post-ictal automatisms', meaning after a seizure) are sometimes used to describe behaviour after a seizure, such as taking a walk or going to bed – the person may look purposeful but has in fact no awareness of what they are doing, and will have no recollection of it afterwards.

Some people suffer confusion and irritability after seizures, together with memory loss not just for the seizure but sometimes for events just before. Headache and tiredness, sometimes extreme, are other common reactions. Some people may also experience weakness, especially down one side of the body.

Nocturnal seizures

The brain is more susceptible to developing seizures during sleep, and some people only have seizures when asleep or dozing. These are called nocturnal seizures, even though they may occur during daytime sleep as well. The positive aspect of nocturnal seizures is that people who have seizures only during sleep may experience fewer restrictions on employment and driving. Sometimes seizures in sleep may be reduced by increasing the evening dosage of anti-epileptic medication, though this should only be done under your doctor's guidance.

Status epilepticus – when it becomes an emergency

Most seizures last only a short time, around 1–3 minutes, and rarely need medical help. A prolonged seizure, however, is a medical emergency.

Status epilepticus, Latin for 'state of epilepsy', is the name given to a continuous prolonged seizure lasting for at least 30 minutes, or a series of seizures that occur in succession for 30 minutes or more, when the person does not recover consciousness between seizures. When seizures go on for up to 5 minutes without signs of stopping, it is possible that status epilepticus may be developing, so that it is generally advised to seek emergency medical help after 5 minutes; or if the person does not recover consciousness; or if the seizure is longer than normal, or seems different in some way to its usual pattern. Generally, seizures which continue for longer than 5–10 minutes need treatment as soon as possible.

The threat of status epilepticus is usually held over your head if you discontinue anti-epileptic medicine, but what are the risks really? Although epilepsy rarely causes brain damage, convulsive status epilepticus (a progression of generalized tonic-clonic seizures) may cause brain damage and occasionally death in up to 10 per cent of people, though prompt medical treatment usually prevents this. Recent evidence suggests that it is not the seizures themselves but the cause of the seizures that may do the damage, such as meningitis, encephalitis or brain tumour. Sometimes status may happen as a first seizure, and in this case, it is often a first and only seizure.

Other types of prolonged seizures, such as prolonged generalized (such as absence) or partial seizures are less immediately dangerous in that they are less likely to cause brain damage, but should still be treated urgently. This type of non-convulsive status can rarely develop into the more dangerous convulsive kind.

Treatment consists of injecting anti-epileptic drugs such as diazepam. Status epilepticus is also sometimes related to not taking anti-epileptic drugs, and is a major reason why it is so important to take medication regularly and not to try and withdraw from anti-epileptic drugs without medical supervision.

The other occasion when you should summon medical help is in a first seizure, particularly if the seizure lasts more than around ten minutes, though most people will do this automatically.

Epilepsy syndromes

One reason why doctors need to differentiate and classify different types of seizures is that sometimes these build into a recognizable syndrome. A syndrome is when certain symptoms occur together to form an identifiable medical condition. Recognizing different syndromes is in turn important because it can give a more accurate idea of the best treatment, and of the prognosis, or long-term outlook.

As well as the type of seizure, doctors need to know the age at which seizures began (many syndromes begin and/or end at certain ages), as well as a person's general developmental or learning abilities. An EEG may also show up certain typical patterns. Some epilepsy syndromes have been identified; and many other syndromes which affect neurological function also include epilepsy. However, only around half of all people with epilepsy will be found to have a clear-cut epilepsy syndrome. Some syndromes are serious, and with a poor outlook, but these are thankfully quite rare.

Two more common and relatively mild syndromes are Benign Rolandic Epilepsy of Childhood (BREC), which is usually outgrown by age 13–16, and juvenile myoclonic epilepsy (JME), which is thought to have a genetic cause, and which often begins in adolescence and is easily controlled.

Two much more rare and serious syndromes are West Syndrome, and the Lennox-Gastaut Syndrome – the first one, which affects babies, often develops into the second. West Syndrome (infantile spasms or salaam spasms) usually begins during the first year of life, and may be caused by developmental brain problems or brain damage. Lennox-Gastaut Syndrome (minor motor epilepsy or slow spike-wave epilepsy) typically involves frequent, hard-to-control seizures, and learning difficulties and development problems.

Gender differences in seizures and syndromes

Some types of seizure are more common in girls and women. At least 60 per cent of children who suffer absence seizures (childhood absence epilepsy) are girls, and recent research suggests there is probably a genetic reason.

Photosensitive epilepsy is twice as common in women as in men (see below under seizure triggers). Hormonal factors have been suggested as a reason but it is more likely that genetic influences are responsible.

A few very rare epilepsy syndromes only affect girls. For example, in Rett Syndrome baby girls appear normal for about the first year, but then start to suffer developmental delay and mental retardation along with epilepsy which is usually hard to control. Aicardi Syndrome, which involves infantile spasms and severe mental retardation, is thought to be a disorder of the X chromosome.

Some syndromes are more common in boys. For example, more boys than girls suffer from West Syndrome (around three boys to two girls).

Seizure triggers

Julie found that her attacks seemed to coincide with being asked about her condition and in fact had a seizure in the shower shortly after completing a questionnaire for this book!

Anthea's seizures included stress at work, disagreements with her family, not getting enough sleep, missing meals, menstruation and too much alcohol – all relatively common triggers of seizures.

Sometimes, seizures can be triggered by certain environmental or internal factors, which can sometimes be quite individual and idiosyncratic. Both Julie and Anthea, like many other people with epilepsy, found that personal stress in its different forms brought on seizures. Seizure triggers are often individual but in general include:

- Stress – the key trigger for many. This includes strong emotions such as fear, anger and excitement; emotional upset or confrontations; and the pressure of work or financial difficulties. Stress can affect areas such as diet, sleep and general health, which can all combine to lower your seizure threshold. Some people have found they also have seizures after a period of stress such as leaving work to go on holiday.
- Lack of sleep – sleep is known to change the brain's patterns of electrical activity, and lack of it can trigger seizures.
- Not taking medication – a surprisingly common seizure trigger. There are many reasons why people don't take their drugs, including forgetfulness, rebellion, and being pregnant and not wanting to harm the unborn baby.
- General health – a person who is unwell may be more likely to have a seizure as overall resistance is lowered. A high temperature may also make some people more prone to seizures. And, illness which includes vomiting and/or diarrhoea will affect absorption of anti-epileptic drugs.
- Menstruation – some women find that their seizures increase around the time of their period ('catamenial epilepsy', further explained in Chapter 5).
- Alcohol – too much alcohol can trigger seizures in some, and some anti-epileptic medication may also make a person more sensitive to its effects.
- Boredom – research has shown that someone who is enjoyably occupied is less likely to have a seizure.
- Lights, noises and patterns – flashing lights are perhaps the best-known triggers of seizures but in fact only affect around 4 per cent of people with epilepsy. So-called 'photosensitive epilepsy' is a form of reflex epilepsy, when a person reacts with a seizure to specific stimuli, which may include strobe lights, television, videos, computers, flickering sunlight, as well as noises which tend to be

idiosyncratic and individual – people have reported being affected by bells, music, the sound of a central heating system or the whirr of a fan. Reflex epilepsy may also involve seizures triggered by other stimuli, including sequentially moving objects such as a line of traffic, or certain patterns, such as square-patterned lino, stripes in a venetian blind, or even printed words.

- Intense exercise has been reported as a trigger by some.
- Dietary factors – eating regularly is important to maintain overall health and keep blood sugar levels steady; blood sugar levels are often low at the time of a seizure. Some people have found that allergic reactions to certain foods such as sugar and caffeine seem to trigger seizures. Certain nutrient shortages have also been linked with seizures, such as lack of calcium, iron, and vitamins B6 and D.
- Medication may lower seizure threshold, including antidepressants, other drugs used by psychiatrists such as phenothiazines, isoniazid for TB and high doses of penicillin. A few people find that they cannot take certain other preparations, such as cough medicine.

Prodromata and predicting seizures

Two or three days before I have a seizure I get a headache which comes and goes. I see flickering light which obstructs my vision and leaves my eyes bloodshot and tired feeling. My family steer clear of me because, although I'm not really aware of it, I suffer mood swings during the run up to a seizure and am not easy to live with.
Anthea

The run-up to a seizure is known medically as the prodrome or prodromata, and some people with epilepsy are more aware of it than others. Unfortunately, it is usually unpleasant, involving feelings such as depression, irritability and heaviness; less commonly, it may involve feelings of elation or exultation. This prodrome is different from an aura in that it lasts longer, coming on typically several hours or even days before a seizure, while an aura is really the beginning of the seizure itself. The prodrome is thought to be caused by subtle abnormal changes in the electrical activity of the brain which finally build up to a seizure, though another possibility is that it is the moods of irritability and depression which finally provoke the seizure.

Given all this, is it possible for seizures to be predicted? Several research centres are exploring this. For example, researchers at the

University of Bonn analysed EEGs and found that an average 11 minutes before a seizure begins there is a characteristic 'loss of complexity' in brainwaves. The German research team scanned the electrical landscape of the brain before and after seizures using a mathematical property from chaos theory known as 'correlation dimension', a number which acts as a measure of how complex the brain's neural activity is. Researchers in America, headed by the US Department of Energy (DOE), also analysed EEG data and found they could detect a seizure 8 to 15 minutes before it occurred.

Research like this may help scientists develop more sensitive methods to detect and possibly prevent oncoming seizures. This could involve mind control techniques where people could try and prevent a seizure using methods such as distraction (see Chapter 4 for more on this) – the German team are testing whether patients whose seizures originate in the hippocampus, a region associated with memory and learning, can avoid seizures by means of memory or learning tasks. Or, it could involve sophisticated technology, such as an implantable monitor, capable of providing a warning or automatically delivering drugs or electrical stimulation to the brain if a seizure is pending. In practice, however, useful though they would be, such devices remain experimental for the time being.

3

Diagnosis and treatment: anti-epileptic drugs

Every day 100 people are newly diagnosed with epilepsy. If you've been through the diagnostic procedure, or are going through it, you may wonder how this can be so, as the whole procedure can be so complicated and prolonged! However, here are a number of reasons why diagnosis can be prolonged, frustrating though this can be at the time. Apart from anything else, your doctor may hesitate to diagnose epilepsy if there is any doubt because of the implications of the condition, including long-term medication and the possible effects on your life, including driving restrictions.

Is it really epilepsy?

Studies suggest that up to a quarter of epilepsy patients may be misdiagnosed. It goes without saying how serious the consequences can be, with education and employment prospects affected as well as health and social ones. People misdiagnosed with epilepsy have suffered loss of jobs, unemployment or refusal of jobs; loss of driving licence; side effects from unnecessary drugs; and loss of social confidence. Two main causes of misdiagnosis have been highlighted.

- first and foremost, over-interpreting the episode of loss of consciousness, plus failure to take a proper medical history – that is, not getting an accurate eye-witness report of seizures;
- wrong interpretation of the EEG (see below).

This certainly highlights the importance of getting the right medical attention from the start, including if in doubt a second, expert opinion from a neurologist, preferably with a specialist interest in epilepsy. It also shows how much responsibility lies with you and those around you when first going to the doctor. There are many common conditions which can be confused with epilepsy.

Alice, 16, fainted at school after trapping her finger in a door, and was observed to twitch and shake as she lay on the floor. Her teacher, who had just done a course in first aid, was anxious that her

27

parents rush her off to casualty for an EEG to be taken in case epilepsy was in question. Her mother, however, preferred to consult the family doctor first, who told her it was a classic vasovagal attack, or faint, caused by sudden pain (see below).

This kind of story is more common than you might think, and does highlight the importance of not precipitating diagnosis on the basis of an isolated episode, or indeed of a number of episodes if they are not epileptic. Most doctors would probably prefer in any case to wait and monitor the situation for a while before making a definitive diagnosis.

Conditions which may be misdiagnosed as epilepsy include:

- **Fainting (syncopal or vasovagal attacks)**, as described in the case history above, may be caused by sudden pain, a shock, a stomach upset, being too warm, or standing for a long time. They tend to be more common in teenage girls. Confusion with epileptic seizures is often made worse by people around trying to sit the person up – the faint has happened because the brain is momentarily short of blood, which also causes any jerking or twitching. Sitting a person up makes this worse – the head needs to be lowered. Another source of confusion is that the symptoms of some partial seizures may resemble symptoms of a faint. However, in a faint, the person usually goes limp after initial jerking (as opposed to having convulsions or going rigid) and tends to recover more quickly than after a seizure.

- **Migraine** resembles epilepsy in that brainwave patterns may show abnormalities during the attack. Like some seizures, migraine is sometimes preceded by an aura including visual disturbances. However, in migraine the aura tends to last for longer, and the visual disturbances are different – seizures tend to involve flashing lights or hallucinations, while migraine typically involves seeing a halo of bright light around objects or losing all or part of your sight. With migraine there should be no loss of consciousness.

- **Hyperventilation**, or overbreathing, often related to stress or panic, means that the person takes in too much oxygen, causing light headedness, dizziness, tingling and sometimes spasms and blackouts. However, some people's epileptic seizures can be brought on by hyperventilating.

- **Cardiac dysrhythmias** or abnormalities of the heart rate or rhythm

28

can cause sudden shortages of blood to the brain which result in loss of consciousness and jerking.

- **Narcolepsy** involves episodes of suddenly falling asleep anywhere and at any time for 30 seconds to a few minutes.

- **Benign paroxysmal vertigo** is when the room seems to be spinning around people. This quickly passes and, unlike some seizures, leaves no confusion or sleepiness.

- **Paroxysmal choreoathetosis** is a group of very rare conditions caused by severe emotional stress, with symptoms which include strange writhing and twisting movements of the arms and legs.

- **Non-Epileptic Attack Disorder** (NEAD) causes seizures which, although 'real' enough, are not epileptic, and are quite common. This means that they do not involve changes in electrical brain activity, and an EEG taken during one will probably be normal. Sorting out epileptic seizures from non-epileptic attacks (NEAs) can be difficult and may need prolonged EEG (including a video record) monitoring as well as psychological treatment such as ignoring seizures and rewarding seizure-free behaviour. NEAs tend to result from psycho-logical factors, such as severe anxiety, stress and post-traumatic stress, but are not under conscious control; some people too have both epileptic and non-epileptic seizures.

  NEAs are generally agreed to be much more common in women than in men. This is not because women are more 'hysterical' but for a complex blend of reasons. Emotional illness seems to be more common in women than in men, or at least is more socially accepted and sanctioned in women. Also, some forms of NEAs are related to previous sexual abuse, which is much more common in women.

- **Transient Ischaemic Attacks** (TIA) are minor strokes lasting less than 24 hours. A TIA tends to involve weakness or numbness, whereas epilepsy tends to involve tingling or jerking of a limb.

- **Transient Global Amnesia** may be relatively common later in life, and is when a person has no memory for a significant period of anything from a few hours up to a day or two. Eyewitnesses say that the person appeared normal and was able to perform complex tasks, though may have often repeated the same question such as 'What time is it?' A person tends to have only a single episode. Transient global amnesia is an important diagnosis because, unlike with epilepsy, people in the UK with this condition, after reporting to the Driver and Vehicle Licensing Agency (DVLA) are allowed to continue driving.

- **Panic attacks** may involve a feeling of fear of an impending event, along with the need to take deep breaths, dizziness, light headedness, and tingling and heaviness in the limbs.

- **Drop attacks** take place for unknown reasons where a middle-aged or older person, often a woman, will suddenly drop to the ground. Consciousness is not lost and the person can get up immediately. There is no treatment.

- **Low blood sugars** (hypoglycaemia) is a rare cause of tonic-clonic seizures, but needs to be excluded in diabetic people on treatment.

- **Alcohol abuse** and withdrawal can sometimes trigger seizures, and certain drugs may do the same.

Diagnosing epilepsy – your medical history

It was not easy to get a diagnosis. My epilepsy seemed to start after a minor car accident and my GP thought I was 'probably not concentrating on my driving'. After a second minor car accident I went to another GP who sent me for further testing including EEG. It took nearly three years to get a proper diagnosis and that was only after I had changed my neurologist with advice from the British Epilepsy Association. In the beginning, it was my husband and myself who were informing the doctors – there is epilepsy in my husband's family and he had been brought up in close touch with it. Counselling, information and support at first were minimal – my first consultant, giving me the results of the tests, said, 'You'll be pleased to know you haven't got a brain tumour', and that was about it! I was asked if I would see a psychiatrist, which I did. He said I definitely didn't need him. My second neurologist was – and is – wonderful. He was the one who told me straight that I had epilepsy, and who bothered to explain what it was.
Julie

As you may already have gathered, diagnosing epilepsy is not always straightforward as even competent doctors can confuse it with several other conditions including psychiatric disorders. What you can tell the doctor may make all the difference and is of prime importance when diagnosing epilepsy. Unless the doctor actually sees a seizure, this isn't a case where he or she can make an intuitive diagnosis based on a glance at the tongue or a feel of the pulse. There is no one test which will detect epilepsy, so what your doctor needs first and foremost is information which only you and those around you can give. This information breaks down into two major parts – an eyewitness account of your seizures, and a detailed medical history covering your past back to babyhood. Because both are so important, it can be a good idea to prepare for both before going to the doctor's, ideally with someone who has seen you have a seizure. This is a situation where it does pay to take responsibility rather than leaving it all to medical carers who are in fact dependent on you for the data which will lead to any treatment.

The eyewitness account

This is extremely important. Epilepsy is peculiar in that it is often impossible for the patient to describe the main symptom, the seizure. Because you do not witness yourself having a seizure, and may be unconscious during the event, it is vital that someone who has seen what has happened can give the doctor an accurate account. It is often difficult to remember exactly what happened – in a first attack in particular everyone is likely to be in a state of shock. It may help to write down as much as possible of what you do remember before going to the doctor. As well as describing the attack in words, the eyewitness could also physically mime what happened. Another idea is to videotape a seizure, or if possible several seizures; it may seem a little cold-blooded for your nearest and dearest to stand around with a camera while you are in the throes of a seizure, but it would certainly help in the interests of accuracy, and does mimic advanced hospital tests which combine video monitoring with other tests.

Your doctor may ask you and whoever accompanies you several questions in order to gain a more complete picture of the attack, such as:

- What happened just before the seizure? This is often the most difficult part to remember, but includes what you were doing, and whether you were in any particular circumstances such as feeling very tired, hungry, thirsty, stressed or angry.
- What time of day did it take place? For example, early morning or at night?
- Did you have any unusual sensations before the attack which might have been a warning (aura), such as a sick, churning feeling in the stomach or a feeling of unusual panic?

31

- Did you have any other symptoms of feeling unwell, such as feeling faint or giddy?
- Were you conscious of the attack or of any details that happened during it?
- How did you feel when you came round?

Your past medical history

This could comprise anything from a difficult birth to heart murmurs at birth or episodes of fainting during childhood. The most relevant past history is febrile convulsions as an infant. It is important not to jump to conclusions, but to mention anything you think might be relevant. Again, because it is quite common to have only a hazy memory of childhood illnesses, you could research this before your visit to the doctor, by asking parents and other relatives what they recall of your birth, and of your health as a baby and child.

As already stated, the most common reason for misdiagnosing epilepsy is that this initial history, perhaps given in something of a panic after a first seizure, is incomplete or wrong. So, don't expect an instant diagnosis.

Diagnostic tests

Referral for hospital tests may take several weeks, which can be frustrating and worrying. However, it is best to be quite sure that epilepsy is in question before making a definite diagnosis. The specialist will probably ask much the same questions as your GP – sometimes an important detail, previously forgotten, may be unearthed by another round of questioning.

The tests you are likely to have include:

Electroencephalography (EEG)

This examines the brain's electrical brainwaves and shows up any abnormal patterns. Sensors called electrodes are placed on the scalp, which transfer the brain activity to the EEG machine where they can be viewed on computer screens or printed out. This process is quite painless.

The limitation of EEGs is that around half of all people with epilepsy show normal brainwave patterns between seizures – and, occasionally, people without epilepsy may show abnormal EEGs. Doctors do have ways of trying to get a clearer result. One is asking you to watch a flashing light to check for photosensitivity, or to breathe deeply as some people have more seizures when hyperventilating. Having less sleep than normal before an EEG is another way, as lack of sleep can sometimes show up abnormal patterns; alternatively, falling asleep during an EEG can sometimes be of value as some patterns show up better during sleep. For this reason you may be asked to stay in hospital overnight, or take away a portable type of EEG called *ambulatory monitoring*. This is EEG monitoring over a period of several hours or sometimes days in which you may walk about and generally get on with your normal activities. Because monitoring lasts longer, it is much more likely to pick up abnormal activity or a seizure. At some centres, an EEG may be done by video – what's called *videotelemetry*. A video camera linked to an EEG machine will put together what any seizures look like, with the electrical evidence from the EEG. This can be done over a period of days, and is often used for people who are being considered for surgery. But, as the equipment is expensive, it is not widely available.

The skull is actually a poor conductor of electricity, which interferes with the transmission of electrical charges to the scalp. Although the brain and the scalp are separated by only a few millimetres, the distance is an enormous chasm in EEG terms. Also, the voltage generated by brain cells and picked up by EEG is extremely small – between 20 and 100 microvolts after amplification on the order of 10,000 times. The signal is so small that electrical interference, called artifacts, from outside sources – for example, motors, overhead lights, even an eye blink – is often as strong as the signal that the EEG is trying to detect. When reading EEG charts, physicians need skill and experience to distinguish artifacts from brain activity and to decode the brain's electrical rhythms into diagnostic information. This is why mistakes in reading an EEG are another common cause of misdiagnosis.

Brain scans

Today's sophisticated scanning techniques give extremely clear and detailed pictures of the brain – but cannot always reveal a cause for the epilepsy. In fact, most people with epilepsy have normal brain scans. However, it is worth having a scan if only to set everyone's mind at rest by excluding structural damage, malformation, or, rarely, tumour. The two main types of scan are CT and MRI. Both involve lying still for 20–45 minutes in a kind of tunnel within the scanning machine. Some people find the idea claustrophobic. However, staff are usually very reassuring and, if you are extremely nervous or have frequent seizures, a light sedative can be given. In fact, more people are troubled by the noise of the MRI machine – staff can also provide earplugs as well as words of support!

- *Computerized axial tomography (CT or CAT)* uses a specialized type of X-ray which takes images of the brain at different angles, using tiny beams of radiation. The pictures are then fed into a computer which comes up with pictures of the brain in 'slices' which, placed together, form a complete view of the brain. If the pictures seem to show something, a special dye is injected via the hand or arm which passes into the body and shows the image more clearly on the scan. CT can show the more obvious sort of brain damage or abnormality such as congenital malformation (i.e., when the brain never developed properly). The test takes around 15–20 minutes.

- *MRI (Magnetic Resonance Imaging)* can give more detailed pictures than CT, using a different technique, magnetism. By bouncing magnetic fields and radio waves (not radiation) off the brain, MRI forms pictures of the brain structure. It may pick up subtle abnormalities or tiny scars or lesions within the brain tissue that CT misses. MRI measures the energy given out by hydrogen atoms within the brain and then creates a picture based on these signals. Its precision also makes it particularly useful as as pre-surgery test (see Surgery, below). The test usually takes around 45 minutes.

PET and SPECT scans

Newer types of scan show how the brain is functioning, as well as giving pictures of its underlying structure. Positron emission tomography (PET) imaging is used to identify areas of the brain which are producing seizures. The images come from radioactive chemicals which are injected into the body and reach the brain, where they concentrate, so showing up specific areas more clearly. Single Photon Emission Computerized Tomography (SPECT) works on the same principle as PET and may take over from it as a more efficient testing tool to show up seizure sources (areas of the brain from which seizures start). However, both are currently used only for research.

Once you've been diagnosed

Alan, who suffered complex partial seizures, knew that something had been wrong for some time but was not really prepared for a diagnosis of epilepsy. He felt that, because he was generally healthy and well, he didn't have a real illness. 'It was more like a sort of shadow I would have to live with for the rest of my life – more real to other people than to me in some ways.' He resented the fact that other people had had power over him, first in terms of witnessing his seizures, and second in diagnosing them, whereas he had only limited experience of the event. He felt vulnerable, and rather afraid of all that epilepsy might imply.

Coming to terms with a diagnosis of epilepsy is not easy. You may feel shocked, or that the doctors have made a mistake. It will not help if you have the brisk kind of GP who considers counselling to consist of telling you that you must now give up your driving licence and wait until you have been seizure-free for 12 months before being able to re-apply – this has happened.

But, you probably need to discuss the diagnosis with your doctor, as there may be aspects of it you don't understand or agree with. It can be hard to take everything in at once, especially if you are in a state of shock at the diagnosis. It is worth getting the facts as clear as possible right from the outset, as many people feel rather half-hearted about asking basic facts once they are enrolled in the medical system and installed on medication. Diagnosis, a key time for finding out about your epilepsy, is often missed by people. One survey by the British Epilepsy Association showed that as many as one third of patients with epilepsy did not know what type of epilepsy they had. So, now is the time to ask questions, either of your GP, an epilepsy specialist, or, if you have access to one at your treatment centre, an epilepsy nurse specialist who is expert at understanding the particular concerns of the time. You are bound to think of questions you want to ask after your initial doctor's appointment, so it may help to make a special further appointment to find out what you need to know. You might also find it helpful to contact one of the epilepsy self-help organizations such as the British Epilepsy Association (BEA), or the National Society for Epilepsy (NSE) (see Useful addresses).

Talking with your doctor is also obviously vital if you disagree with your diagnosis and want to challenge it. This can be done at GP or at specialist level. If talking to your usual GP gets you nowhere, you do have the right to a second opinion, either from another GP or – and this may be preferable – from a specialist in epilepsy. Ask your GP to refer you if he or she has not already. If you have talked to a specialist and are still not happy, then it is possible again to seek another opinion at specialist level. Again, you can ask your GP to refer you. It may help if you have a specific idea of where you would like to go for a second opinion, and a national epilepsy self-help group may be able to give you advice about epilepsy centres. Bear in mind that this may mean more weeks or months of waiting, though you may feel it is preferable to remaining in doubt as to whether the diagnosis is right.

Asking questions

You may need time in which to absorb your diagnosis or you may need to know as much as possible straight away. Either way, it is a good idea to find out as much as possible about your epilepsy, medication and any possible side effects – uncertainty causes stress. You may find it helpful to make notes of the answers.

Common questions include:

- Exactly what type of epilepsy do I have?
- What other medications can I take?
- When do I take my tablets?
- What happens if I miss a dose?
- Can I drink?
- What might trigger a seizure?
- Do I need to consider other lifestyle issues such as stress?
- Could I have information about counselling to discuss new lifestyle issues which have arisen, such as a new relationship or bereavement?
- What about pregnancy and breastfeeding?
- Can I drive?
- Can I think about decreasing my medication?
- What should I do if I need to discuss my treatment between appointments?

Research by the British Epilepsy Association has shown that women in particular often feel they are not given enough information, and the BEA suggests the following questions you may want to ask your doctor.

Will my treatment:

- affect my menstrual cycle?
- interfere with my oral contraceptive pill?
- have side effects (e.g. weight gain, unwanted hair growth, tiredness)?
- need to change if I plan to start a family?

- affect my ability to conceive a child?
- affect my unborn child?

Hopefully this book will provide answers to many of these questions – Chapters 5 and 6 in particular look at menstruation, contraception, fertility, family planning and pregnancy.

Sometimes, disagreeing with diagnosis can be part of a difficulty in accepting epilepsy. This takes time, and can be a complex procedure. There's more about epilepsy and your feelings in Chapter 9.

Deciding on treatment

The main form of treatment for epilepsy is drugs, but putting people on to long-term medication is not to be undertaken lightly, both in terms of the financial cost to the health service and, more importantly, the personal cost to you.

This said, many doctors believe that treatment for epilepsy should be started sooner rather than later because it achieves better seizure control, lowers the risk of recurrence if you later come off your drugs, and makes for a better prognosis generally. There is some evidence to show that starting treatment early has some beneficial effect on the course of the epilepsy itself – i.e., it doesn't just stop seizures but may impact on the underlying cause and general brain health – while delaying treatment may make epilepsy worse, and make control harder to achieve later on.

Not all doctors agree. Some question the use of routine prescribing on the grounds that it is not proven that early treatment affects the course of the epilepsy. According to this point of view, epilepsy is a group of conditions, in which responses to drugs will differ. Also, prognosis depends on various unchangeable factors, such as the type of epilepsy, and the age at which it started, which will not be affected by early treatment. Some clinical trials comparing early treatment with deferred treatment did not seem to show any great benefit to earlier treatment. Some studies have shown that epilepsy sometimes seems to remit or stop spontaneously without treatment. For example, an American study of 204 patients reported in the *New England Journal of Medicine* found that only a third of patients who have a single seizure are likely to have any more seizures.

However, this is largely an academic argument, to be thrashed out at consultant level in medical journals; in practice, most doctors would agree that treatment should be started after two tonic-clonic seizures.

Anti-epileptic drugs

Anti-epileptic or anticonvulsant drugs control seizures in up to 80 per cent of all people with epilepsy. In up to 70 per cent, this will be with one drug – monotherapy, which is obviously preferred by both doctors and patients as being simpler and with fewer potential side effects. In around another 10 per cent of people, seizures will be controlled by a combination of two drugs. In the remaining people, seizures will be harder to control, and may involve trial and error with different drugs at different dosages.

Curiously, it isn't known exactly *how* many of the established anti-epileptic drugs work, but they are thought to slow down the tendency of brain cells to fire, or to alter brain chemicals so as to achieve a better balance of electrical activity.

Once the decision to treat has been made, your doctor will decide on the drug of first choice, basing the decision on the type of seizures in question, and balancing how well the drug works (efficacy) against possible side effects.

The ideal aim of drugs is to control seizures with minimal side effects, and doctors usually start at a lower dose and build up, to avoid side effects as much as possible. Regular monitoring assesses the effect of medication, and occasionally with some drugs your doctor may perform blood tests to check drug levels.

Which drugs, which side effects?

Anti-epileptic drugs can be classified into four main types – very old, older, newer and newest. This, while probably not the official medical classification, does reflect the history of drugs for epilepsy, which has had long gaps between new medications. It is only in the last decade that a host of really new drugs have appeared which have been targeted much more precisely at epilepsy – the older ones, designed for other conditions and found incidentally to be useful for epilepsy, tend to work by 'damping down' brain activity in general and can have more side effects.

One very old drug is bromide, the first drug ever to be used for epilepsy, from 1880, and probably to blame for many of the observations made in the nineteenth century about the 'epileptic personality' (more on this in Chapter 9). It is hardly ever used today except in highly specialist circumstances in epilepsy centres. Paraldehyde, another old drug, is also for specialist use, for example to treat status epilepticus.

Phenobarbitone is an older drug which has been in use since before the First World War and tends to have side effects which may affect functions such as behaviour, memory, alertness and concentration; behaviour may also be affected, with irritability and hyperactivity. For this reason it is now rarely prescribed. Phenytoin has been in use since 1938. It is a difficult drug to use and has possibly more side effects than other newer drugs, but it is still commonly prescribed.

Newer drugs such as carbamazepine and sodium valproate, first used in the 1960s and 1970s, have fewer side effects than the older ones, though they still have some. (See Table 1.)

Side effects are a major problem with drugs for some people. This may be dose-related – typical dose-related side effects include drowsiness, lethargy, dizziness, unsteadiness or a skin rash. Side effects may pass off with time as you become accustomed to the drug, but should always be mentioned to your doctor. A few side effects, though very rare, are serious, affecting the skin, liver and bone marrow. Behaviour, moodiness and concentration are other side effects, especially at first and if the dose is too high, so again it is worth discussing this with your doctor who may be able to adjust the dosage.

Some side effects are particularly unacceptable to women, especially in the sensitive teenage years. These include weight gain, where the main culprits are valproate, vigabatrin and, rarely, gabapentin. Phenytoin, if used in childhood, has the unfortunate effect of changing facial appearance, with excess hair growth (hirsutism) and gum overgrowth. Perhaps even more vitally in terms of a woman's long-term future, fertility may be impaired with sodium valproate. And, certain drugs affect the contraceptive pill, making it less effective; these include carbamazepine, phenytoin, phenobarbitone, primidone and topiramate. Perhaps most controversially, certain drugs pose a threat to the unborn baby, including sodium valproate, carbamazepine, phenytoin, primidone and phenobarbitone (see Chapters 5 and 6).

Steroids are occasionally prescribed for some difficult-to-treat epilepsy in the form of corticosteroids in very young babies. These don't always work and have potentially serious side effects, such as high blood pressure, reducing the body's immunity, and weight gain.

The latest drugs, such as vigabatrin, lamotrigine, piracetam, gabapentin, tiagabine and topiramate, are targeted more specifically at epilepsy, and may have fewer side effects, though long-term side effects may not be established.

Table 1 Main anti-epileptic drugs

The following chart provides general information but should not be used in place of individual medical advice – consult your doctor for more information.

First-line drugs

CARBAMAZEPINE
For: Generalized tonic-clonic and partial seizures.
Side effects: Skin rash, double vision, dizziness, unsteadiness, confused thinking and nausea may occur initially or if the dose is too high. Teratogenic (i.e. can cause problems in baby development during pregnancy). Also interacts with the contraceptive pill, making it less effective.

ETHOSUXIMIDE
For: Absences.
Side effects: Nausea, headache, drowsiness, and very rarely, rash, blood problems and liver diseases.

LAMOTRIGINE
(not for under 16s)
For: Partial and generalized tonic-clonic.
Side effects: Skin rash, Stevens-Johnson syndrome (severe, potentially life-threatening rash), drowsiness, double vision, dizziness and headache.

PHENYTOIN
For: Generalized tonic-clonic and partial seizures.
Side effects: Skin rash, drowsiness, unsteadiness and slurred speech may occur if the dose is too high. May affect behaviour and learning, and cause decreased energy and alertness. Coarsening of facial features, increased body hair (hirsutism), gum overgrowth and acne with prolonged therapy. May, rarely, affect liver or bone marrow. Teratogenic (i.e. can cause problems in baby development during pregnancy). Also interacts with the contraceptive pill, making it less effective.

SODIUM VALPROATE
For: Generalized tonic-clonic and partial seizures and absences.
Side effects: Drowsiness and tremor are infrequent side effects. Hair loss, which is reversible. Very rarely, liver damage. Teratogenic (i.e. can cause problems in baby development during pregnancy).

Second-line drugs

ACETAZOLOMIDE
For: Generalized tonic-clonic, partial seizures and atypical absences.
Side effects: Lack of appetite, loss of weight, drowsiness, depression, pins and needles in hands and feet, joint pains, increased urine output, thirst, headache, dizziness, fatigue and irritability.

CLOBAZAM
For: Generalized tonic-clonic and partial seizures.
Side effects: Drowsiness.

CLONAZEPAM
For: Partial seizures, absences and myoclonic jerks.
Side effects: Drowsiness and sedation.

GABAPENTIN
For: Partial seizures.
Side effects: Drowsiness, dizziness, headache and fatigue.

PHENOBARBITONE
For: Generalized tonic-clonic and partial seizures.
Side effects: Drowsiness, sedation and mental slowness. Teratogenic (i.e. can cause problems in baby development during pregnancy). Also interacts with the contraceptive pill, making it less effective.

PIRACETAM
For: Myoclonic seizures.
Side effects: Very rare but may include weight gain, diarrhoea, insomnia, drowsiness, nervousness, depression and rash.

PRIMIDONE

For: Generalized tonic-clonic and partial seizures.
Side effects: Nausea, unsteadiness, drowsiness, sedation and mental slowness.

TOPIRAMATE

For: Partial seizures.
Side effects: Mental slowing, weight loss, ataxia, risk of kidney stones, impaired concentration, confusion, dizziness, fatigue, pins and needles, and drowsiness. Appears to be teratogenic and interacts with the contraceptive pill.

VIGABATRIN

For: Partial and secondary generalized seizures.
Side effects: Drowsiness, nausea, and behaviour and mood changes. Psychotic reactions, anxiety and depression.

New drugs

These include **tiagabine**, **oxcarbazepine** and **levoreticam**.

Tiagabine appears affective in people with complex partial seizures, particularly those who have responded to vigabatrin. At the moment it appears from clinical trials to have fewer side effects than vigabatrin.

Oxcarbazepine is a drug related to carbamazepine, but it is broken down differently by the body and so may have much lower side effects, which means that higher doses can be used to treat more resistant epilepsy.

Levoreticam is a new drug that appears to be effective in people with all kinds of epilepsies. Its main side effect appears to be sleepiness.

Drugs of the future seem to have fantastic possibilities. For example, researchers in California have found that the venom of one of the world's biggest spiders, the Cameroon Red Baboon, protects mice against seizures. The extract, code-named SNZ-482, is the first substance known to block a molecule implicated in epilepsy and may help detect causes of epilepsy and test new drugs! This is just one of many compounds. Hard-to-control epilepsy especially is an area where, as might be expected, there is a great deal of scientific interest, given that 20–30 per cent of people will have trouble controlling seizures with drugs.

Problems with drugs

Drugs can work very well for many people with epilepsy, allowing them to lead full and normal lives. Others find medication less easy, either because of side effects or simply because it doesn't work. While many drugs do take a while to be effective, the fact remains that up to 30 per cent of people with epilepsy do not respond to drug therapy. If the drugs do prove ineffective, your doctor may try a higher dose, or a different drug, or a combination of two drugs.

Very rarely anti-epileptic drugs can result in more frequent seizures. If this happens your doctor may check the diagnosis. Doctors usually start patients with epilepsy off on the lowest anti-epileptic dose and then build it up in order to minimize side effects. How much you need depends on various factors such as your build and metabolism, which influence how your body processes the drugs and how easy your epilepsy is to treat.

Too high a dose can result in intoxication. Symptoms of intoxication vary from drug to drug. If someone receives too much phenytoin, they often become very unsteady and can have more frequent seizures. Carbamazepine toxicity usually begins with double vision and drowsiness. Another reason why drugs may sometimes seem to increase seizures is if a drug suitable for one type of seizure aggravates other seizure types. Carbamazepine, for example, is effective against tonic-clonic seizures, but not against absence seizures.

There has also been some confusion over branded versus generic drugs. Nearly all drugs have two names. The first name is the *generic* one, the scientific name given to a drug which is internationally recognized. *Branded* drugs are those with a name created by an individual pharmaceutical company which has manufactured them. The actual drug is the same, but problems can arise if you switch from one to the other – for example, if you go from Tegretol (brand) to carbamazepine (generic). This is because there are sometimes differences in the way the drug was manufactured. It is best that you stick to the type of epilepsy tablets you were initially prescribed, whether branded or generic. Occasionally changing can precipitate seizures or side effects. Conversely occasionally someone's seizure control can improve or side effects decrease.

Changing drug treatment

Before treatment is changed various questions need to be considered:

1 **Is this epilepsy?** The misdiagnosis rate is estimated to be between 10 and 25 per cent.
2 **If it is epilepsy, what is the type of seizure disorder or syndrome?** Many people with juvenile myoclonic epilepsy (tonic-clonic seizures and myoclonic jerks first thing in the morning) go undiagnosed, as relevant leading questions have not been asked about myoclonic jerks or early morning tonic-clonic seizures. This particular syndrome responds extremely well to sodium valproate, but carbamazepine can make seizures worse.
3 **Are you on an appropriate anti-epileptic drug?** All anti-epileptic drugs appear equally effective (or ineffective!) for partial seizures, but in primary and symptomatic generalized epilepsy seizures respond best to sodium valproate, with lamotrigine as second-line therapy.
4 **Is the drug being given in an adequate dosage?** It is amazing how many people are on more than one drug, all the drugs being in inadequate dosages. Results of a clinical audit undertaken in London suggested that seizures could be halved in about a third of people by reducing the number of drugs down to monotherapy and giving that drug in adequate dosage. Interestingly 10 per cent became seizure-free as a result of this simple manoeuvre.
5 **Are you taking the medication?** If this is a problem it is worth trying to simplify therapy to one drug given a maximum of twice a day. The midday dose is very easy to forget and all but gabapentin have a long enough half-life for them to be given either once or twice daily.

If reassessing all the above proves unsuccessful then adding in a second anti-epileptic drug needs consideration, or possibly surgery as an alternative means of therapy.

Stopping drug treatment

Once seizures have been controlled for a while, you may wonder whether it is possible to stop taking medication. There is around a 40 per cent chance of seizures returning if drug treatment is stopped, but unfortunately there is no way of knowing for sure which particular individuals will be affected, though doctors may be able to make an informed guess depending on your type of epilepsy.

The most likely forms of epilepsy to respond well to treatment are juvenile myoclonic epilepsy (JME) and the related syndrome of tonic-clonic seizures on awakening. JME consists of someone having tonic-clonic seizures within two hours of awakening, plus, if leading questions are asked, a history of sudden jerks.

Seizure return is more likely with certain types of seizure, including myoclonic, atonic, tonic and partial seizures, as well as West Syndrome and Lennox-Gastaut Syndrome. Total control is incredibly rare. Research has also shown that other factors increase the risk of recurrence, including a known cause for the epilepsy, seizures which began after age 12, a family history of epilepsy, and a history of atypical febrile seizure, and an abnormal EEG. Other research has found that the longer the seizure-free interval before withdrawal, and the fewer drugs needed for initial seizure control, the greater the likelihood of successful remission.

Your doctor may agree that you could try drug withdrawal after five years of being seizure-free (one to two years if a child). This has to be a calculated risk, bearing in mind the implications for matters such as career and driving. Drugs will be tapered off gradually, with the dosage reduced over a three-to-six-month period. It is important that you adhere faithfully to this doctor-monitored reduction, and that you don't try and 'come off' the drugs yourself. Suddenly stopping medication can be dangerous as it may lead to status epilepticus (a prolonged seizure described in Chapter 2).

If seizures do return, they normally do so relatively soon, within a few weeks or months, and are usually the same kind as before. Some figures show that 50 per cent of seizures which return do so within six months of stopping medication, 60–80 per cent within a year, and virtually all within two years. If seizures do recur, total control on restarting anti-epileptic drugs therapy is likely.

4

Other treatment options

While drugs are the main treatment for epilepsy, there are other options which can be explored if your epilepsy proves resistant to treatment, or if you find drug side effects unacceptable, or if you want to consider other kinds of treatment because, for example, you're planning to become pregnant. While the more precise use of drugs, or a change of drugs, might solve problems for some, there will always be some people whose epilepsy remains hard to control, who suffer disabling side effects from drugs, or who just dislike having to take regular medication.

These other treatments vary enormously, from the highest of high-tech surgical techniques, to the very specialized high-fat ketogenic diet, to the more homely sounding trained dogs who can give warning of seizures. While some of these treatments may have a limited application, either because they're not widely available, or because they may only suit certain forms of epilepsy, epilepsy is an area where the latest research is constantly challenging ideas about the condition. Sometimes, what seemed almost impossible yesterday becomes reality today, such as laser surgery for epilepsy. So, although such treatments may not benefit everyone, they may certainly be worth exploring if you find that drugs do not suit you.

The case for surgery

Susie, 22, at first refused to think about surgery when it was suggested to her. But, an appointment with a specialist neurosurgeon changed her mind as the latest techniques were explained to her along with the risks and benefits of surgery. Her epilepsy, which she'd had from childhood, had been getting steadily worse over the past two years. Previously, her seizures had been mainly nocturnal and had given her enough warning to seek safety, but they now struck increasingly by day, and without any aura. Her confidence and social life were dwindling, and her work as a secretary was becoming almost impossible. Surgery seemed the only option. The operation was a success, though recovery was slow – it took almost a year before she stopped having headaches. Today, however, three years on, she is almost 'cured' of her epilepsy, the only remaining

46

part of her seizures being the aura, and she has been able to withdraw from her medication.

Epilepsy surgery, traditionally the last resort of the person with hard-to-control epilepsy, can seem like a frightening option at first. But, it has aroused new interest and controversy lately as modern neuroimaging techniques make for more accurate diagnosis, while revolutionary electronic and laser methods result in safer surgery. Many doctors now believe that surgery should be used more, and earlier.

Epilepsy surgery is different from drug treatment in that it can actually cure epilepsy, although only a minority of people with epilepsy – around 4–5 per cent – have the type of epilepsy which is currently considered suitable for this treatment. Surgery can be performed if there is an identifiable epileptic zone or abnormality in the brain from which seizures start, something which may be shown on the MRI scan. People may also be considered for surgery if they have frequent, disabling seizures which do not respond to medication, and which are always partial or focal, that is, starting on one side of the brain.

However, new research is expanding the parameters of those considered to be suitable candidates for surgery. For example, a recent study of 2,200 patients in Paris found that mesial temporal lobe epilepsy, which does not respond well to medication but is curable with surgery, is more common than suspected, which means that there may potentially be many thousands of people who would benefit from surgery who are currently not even screened for surgery. Around 80–90 per cent of people with this type of epilepsy, caused by often subtle abnormalities in the brain's hippocampus, will become seizure-free after surgery.

There is also growing recognition that the earlier surgery is performed, the better the likely outcome for the person, not just directly in terms of seizure control, but indirectly in terms of relationships with others, education, employment prospects and other lifestyle issues. This obviously has particular relevance for children, and it has been found that even young babies can be successfully treated by surgery. An American study of 136 operations performed at the Opportunities Cleveland Clinic Foundation in Cleveland, Ohio, showed that nearly 70 per cent of operations led to complete seizure freedom, with an additional 10–20 per cent resulting in substantial improvement and only rare seizures after the operation. This study, reported in the *Annals of Neurology*, the official journal of the American Neurological Association, dealt with young children and adolescents who had previously suffered dozens or even hundreds of seizures a day which had proved resistant to multiple trials of anti-epileptic medication.

One reason why surgery may not be more frequently prescribed is the time and the difficulty in assessing patients for surgery. There are only a few centres able to do assessments for surgery in the UK. Many doctors argue that surgery is ultimately more cost-effective than allowing patients to spend a lifetime as consumers of healthcare resources such as anti-epileptic drugs, routine hospital visits and emergency treatment after injury from seizures. People facing the prospect of an operation may well be more concerned with the risks and benefits than the expense, however, so just what are the success rates and dangers of epilepsy surgery? Success rates vary from centre to centre, but, in general, operations on the temporal lobe have the best chance of success – following anterior temporal lobectomy, some 70 per cent of people are seizure-free and 85–90 per cent show worthwhile improvement, although some people may still have auras or take medication.

Like any other surgery, epilepsy surgery does have its risks, though the main risks are generally considered to be very low (1–2 per cent), and are to do with stroke, paralysis, speech problems, and risks common to all operations such as anaesthetic complication and infection. Candidates for surgery are rigorously screened, and given a battery of exhaustive neuropsychological tests to make sure surgery will not affect vital brain areas, such as language, memory, concentration, motor, visual-spatial and other skills – all particularly important when considering operations within the temporal lobe which is implicated in so many of these functions. Surgery candidates will also undergo other tests such as repeated EEG monitoring, sometimes overnight or longer by videotelemetry, and, rarely, using more invasive electrodes, *depth electrodes*, fine silver needles which penetrate the skull to the brain in order to monitor epileptic activity more precisely. CT scans and MRI scans will also be needed. None of this is done quickly, especially as you may have to wait for an appointment at a specialist epilepsy centre, rather than an ordinary hospital. It may be a year or longer before all tests are completed and an operation is carried out.

Epilepsy surgery works by removing the source of the seizures, such as a scar, when it's known as *resective surgery*. Alternatively, surgery may involve disconnecting the seizure source (part of the brain from which seizures start) from other parts of the brain (*disconnection surgery*). This is done by cutting nerve fibres so that seizure activity can no longer travel along the nerve pathways. Disconnection surgery interferes with the spread of a seizure, but doesn't remove the part of the brain which causes a seizure. New methods of surgery are also becoming available and have aroused a great deal of interest, although like other surgery their use is limited, as the next sections explain.

The gamma knife

Publicity about the laser gamma knife has caused a great deal of interest, and this is indeed a highly sophisticated and precise technique, though still in its infancy. Early results indicate it can be a very effective form of treatment, with 70–75 per cent of patients having the severity and frequency of seizures reduced, though this area is still under research. With the gamma knife, the risks of conventional surgery are minimized, as not only are scanning and computer techniques used to target the area with maximum precision, but the laser means that the skull is not opened at all. Thus, gamma-knife surgery is non-invasive as well as being minutely planned. Suitable patients are those in whom surgery to the temporal lobe might be useful.

However, there are provisos, one of the main ones being that gamma-knife treatment is still a form of surgery, so that the stringent conditions outlined above still apply. It is also still under research, though becoming more available. Most research so far has looked at temporal lobe epilepsy, with the knife being used mainly to treat brain tumours and venous (vein) malformations.

As with conventional surgery, MRI scans help establish the precise area to be targeted. Once the person has been established as being suitable for surgery, the operation itself can take under two hours – around an hour and a half for treatment planning, and the operation itself from around 20 minutes.

The gamma knife works by using very high doses of radiation, which are targeted very specifically at tiny areas of the brain such as malformations and tumours. Many small rays are aimed at the target, and there is just one session – the treatment doesn't have to be repeated. This method of surgery, known as radiosurgery, can use up to 50 or more greys (units of radiation) in contrast to radiotherapy, which uses maybe 1.5–2.5 greys. Unlike radiotherapy, though, which radiates all cells including 'good' ones, radiosurgery is very precisely aimed at a small area. The patient remains conscious throughout, and usually local anaesthetic only is used to help fit a special frame onto the head which directs the rays. A general anaesthetic is only used with uncontrollable or frequent seizures.

Gamma-knife surgery is sometimes confused with LINAC surgery, surgery using linear accelerators, when radiation is also used, but the rays are delivered differently. LINAC surgery uses only one beam in contrast to the many small rays of gamma-knife surgery, and uses only 10–12 greys, a method which some doctors consider both less effective and more risky.

There are over 100 knives worldwide and over 100,000 patients have been treated with it. Following a French study of 12 patients, research is now being planned by Cromwell Hospital and Sheffield's Royal Hallamshire Hospital, and gamma-knife surgery may be obtained on the NHS at the latter. To find out more, consult your doctor, specialist epilepsy nurse if you have access to one, and contact the Gamma-knife Surgery Support Organization if you or your doctor require more information (addresses at the back of this book).

Vagal Nerve Stimulation (VNS)

VNS is a form of stimulation of the brain which seems to improve epilepsy in some people and involves implanting a small device rather like a pacemaker in the person's chest (hence this too is classified as surgery). A major study carried out at several international medical centres, and reported in the journal *Neurology*, found that patients had their seizures reduced by nearly a third, and concluded that VNS is here to stay as a valid, safe epilepsy treatment. Other estimates of its success rate have found an even more encouraging 50 per cent reduction in seizure frequency, with some people being able to reduce medication. However, as these figures imply, it doesn't work for everyone, and it may also take time to work – an estimated three to six months.

Following extensive research which revealed that brainwave patterns changed when the vagus nerve was stimulated, vagal nerve stimulation was first applied by Dr Jacob Zabara, a neurophysiologist at Temple University, Philadelphia, USA. The method involves mild electrical stimulation of the vagus nerve which carries information to the brain. While it isn't known exactly how this helps control seizures, it is thought that some of the nerves in the vagus nerve have connections to areas of the brain involved in producing seizures, and that the electric signals interrupt or disconnect this activity. The VNS device is implanted in the upper left chest during a one-to-three-hour operation.

Once implanted, the device is usually set to fire at regular intervals (such as 30 times a second for 30 seconds every 300 seconds) but can be adjusted according to individual need in the weeks following the operation by means of an external computer programme. Regular appointments continue after programming is completed, and patients are usually asked to complete a seizure diary card to monitor how VNS is affecting the seizures. Some people who feel a seizure coming on between programmed doses can also use a small magnet to make the device fire themselves, by placing the magnet over the generator for about two seconds; if you are having a seizure, someone else can do the same.

Side effects are usually said to be mild and transient, though the generator leaves a bulge on the upper left chest area. The main side effects are tingling in the neck, hoarseness, coughing, voice alteration, shortness of breath, throat pain, and ear or tooth pain. Altering the stimulation level can help alleviate these if they don't pass spontaneously. In a very few people, the device may increase seizures, and if this happens it can be turned off using the magnet again.

VNS may be available on the NHS – ask your doctor, specialist epilepsy nurse, or contact the support group FABLE (For a Better Life with Epilepsy – see Useful addresses).

Mind control techniques

The psychological component of seizures is widely recognized, with many people having more seizures when angry or upset. At its most negative, this can easily become a stick to beat yourself with: 'I must have a quiet life.' It can also be used by others: 'You must have a quiet life!' On the positive side, it can be used to advantage in that some people may be able to train themselves out of having seizures. Research at London's Maudsley Hospital has estimated that around a third of people can sometimes stop seizures using mental techniques. One study of people with difficult-to-control epilepsy found that, using self-control methods as well as their usual medication, they could reduce their seizures drastically – 68 per cent managed an 80–100 per cent reduction, and 12 per cent had a 60–70 per cent reduction of seizures.

The training fell into three main parts which are common to many mind control techniques:

- helping people identify the warning signals of a seizure;
- helping people identify factors likely to trigger a seizure (such as strong stress);
- helping people develop counter measures to ward off a seizure, including distraction methods and learning how to relax.

Some people learn to do this spontaneously.

> Anthea would recite the two-times table as a form of distraction if she felt a seizure coming on. If the aura was gradual, Bronwen could sometimes make it subside by focusing on an object in the room such as a piece of clothing on the floor, and forcing herself to get up and put it away. Alan would brush his teeth, and also found music helpful to listen to as it helped to concentrate his mind.

Obviously, this kind of treatment is only going to work if you have some kind of warning of seizures, that is, if you have partial seizures or secondarily generalized seizures that begin with some kind of warning or aura, so that you have time to take action. Some people also have typical pre-seizure moods (see the section on prodrome, Chapter 2), so that if you don't recognize your pre-seizure mood yourself, you could ask family or friends to warn you. Keeping a seizure diary is a good way of recognizing seizure triggers, again perhaps with the help of a friend or partner, and there's more on how to keep a diary in Chapter 7.

One of the main forms of mind control techniques is biofeedback, which is really a kind of reward therapy – the reward being the 'feedback' which comes as visible or audible proof of how well a person is controlling the brain's electrical activity. Biofeedback acts on the principle that it is easier to gain awareness and control of physical processes if we can see or hear the 'feedback'. Biofeedback uses various instruments to measure the information the body is giving out, and convert it into a readable signal such as a light or bleep. Biofeedback for epilepsy uses EEG to measure brain activity, which may then be shown as a computer image which the person has the power to change using mental techniques which also control brain activity. This has around a 33 per cent success rate, according to Dr Peter Fenwick, consultant at the Institute of Psychiatry, London, and leader of much research into epilepsy and biofeedback. German and American studies have also found that people were able to lower seizure frequency and strength significantly after 20–25 sessions of biofeedback training.

Alternative therapies

Often in a less structured way, the elements of mind control can play an important part in many alternative therapies. Just by feeling more relaxed, people can often ward off a seizure; or they may consciously use them as distraction. Alternative therapies can also be very helpful in giving people a sense of control over their own lives, their treatment and their epilepsy.

Certain aromatherapy oils such as ylang ylang, lavender and camomile are usually viewed as relaxing, which together with a soothing massage may be enough to ward off a seizure. Aromatherapy is also one of the few alternative therapies which has come under scientific scrutiny. Patients in Birmingham University's Seizure Clinic were asked to choose an oil that appealed to them and if necessary were taught to relax using massage with this oil. They were then taught to associate feeling relaxed with the smell of the oil in order to create a kind of protective memory cache to dip into at times of stress when a seizure seemed to be pending. By creating a memory link between the smell of the oil and the state of relaxation, smelling the oil at a later date would help people recall feeling relaxed. Patients also learned to use self-hypnosis or visualization techniques which remind them of the relaxing 'smell memory' of the oil, and the relaxed state it evoked. It's thought that the smell of the oils works on the olfactory (smell) centres in the temporal lobes of the brain, which in turn affect the brain's limbic area, involved in the senses, mood control, instinctive behaviour, and emotions.

Audits of the results of using this specialized form of aromatherapy have been encouraging and do suggest that some people (if they practise and if they have the right kind of epilepsy with the right kind of warnings) can use this technique as a self-control measure. A few patients have been able to lose their seizures. Once learned, the technique seems to continue to be effective. The unit is currently researching an observation that possibly one or two aromatherapy oils, particularly jasmine, may have anti-epilepsy properties; this research is in its very early stages.

However, there is no reason why you could not benefit from the relaxing effects of aromatherapy massage. Just be aware that some aromatherapy oils are thought to stimulate the brain and seizure activity and should be avoided by people with epilepsy – they include hyssop, rosemary, sweet fennel and sage. Rosemary, for example, contains camphor, a convulsant which was used – apparently successfully – in the seventeenth century in Switzerland, England and Germany to treat mania by producing convulsions. If you do visit an aromatherapist, make sure she or he knows you have epilepsy.

Other remedies which have been tried by people with epilepsy include acupuncture (with acupressure and shiatsu), Traditional Chinese Herbal Medicine (TCHM), herbal and homeopathic remedies, and reflexology. While there is very little scientific evidence to support these as remedies, anecdotal evidence suggests that some people find them beneficial, though cost may be a limiting factor, and it is important to check a practitioner's qualifications as far as possible. Always inform a practitioner that you have epilepsy, and never discontinue anti-epileptic drugs on a practitioner's advice without your usual doctor's supervision.

Seizure-alert dogs

One to two hours before a seizure, Sally's dog Rocky begins to behave in an unusual way, circling round, whining and blocking her movements, or perhaps nudging her, pulling at her sleeve, or jumping up. If she takes no notice, the dog becomes more insistent until she realizes what he is trying to tell her: another seizure is on the way. According to Sally, her neurologist has no trouble accepting that this is true, as the bruises and cuts from her seizures have been so markedly reduced.

There are many anecdotes of dogs being able to tell when a seizure is on the way, typically up to an hour or so in advance. Dogs vary in how they convey the message, with individual alert patterns of barking, licking or trying to nudge their owner to safety. Some of these animals are pets, but others are said to be specially trained to detect seizures, called seizure-alert dogs – something like guide dogs for the blind.

While this area is being increasingly researched both in the UK and the US, it is still not clear how the dogs work. It may be that they can sense changes in the brain which precede a seizure, or very subtle shifts in attention, behaviour or mood long before they become evident to humans. It has also been suggested that people may undergo subtle changes in odour caused by chemical changes in the body just before a seizure, which might be picked up by a dog's keen sense of smell.

Although there are anecdotal reports of dogs responding spontaneously to seizures, dogs which become seizure-alert dogs do need to be properly and humanely trained. There has been some concern about training dogs to be exposed to potentially distressing events like seizures. But, dog trainers believe that the dogs will only suffer fear and stress if repeatedly exposed to seizures without specialist training. Specialist training, properly done, is not distressing for the dog, who is allowed its full complement of play, exercise and attention. While most breeds can be used, trainers may look for specific qualities in the puppy, such as being very aware of their surroundings, but not too easily distracted by them. The dogs need to be devoted, loyal, dependable and highly obedient, and above all, enjoy working and being with people.

A number of institutions exist which claim to train animals as seizure-alert dogs, and these are coming up for some serious research both in the UK and in the US. In the UK, Support Dogs, in Sheffield, a charity which depends on outside contributions for the £1,500 cost of training each dog, is involved in a research project with the David Lewis Centre for Epilepsy and also in research with leading neurologist Dr Stephen Brown. This project will measure the effects of seizure-alert dogs on quality of life for people with epilepsy.

Neurologists at the University of Florida are looking at whether the ability to detect seizures is a spontaneous reaction or a trainable behaviour, and are studying not just anecdotal evidence from people who say they have such dogs, but also the groups that claim to be able to train them. Some of the training groups make more aggressive claims than others, and different organizations have varying degrees of success. At the moment, few dogs are trained and certified, though this may change with more research, knowledge and funding.

The function of seizure-alert dogs can go well beyond warning of impending seizures. By offering protection as well as guidance, they can open up a whole new way of life for certain people with epilepsy. Sally, mentioned above, had been virtually housebound through fear of seizures, but felt much less vulnerable with a dependable dog. The dog may protect its owner in many ways – anecdotes exist of dogs protecting their owners from robbery while they were vulnerable during a seizure in a public place. They may have a special role with complex partial seizures which are not obvious to others, when the person may need protection or guidance back to a safe environment.

Dogs may also make a difference to those who previously lacked confidence to try for a job. Having a seizure-alert dog may also be reassuring for employers, who might otherwise hesitate to employ a person through fear of unpredictable seizures. As with so many other areas of epilepsy, employers may well need to be educated about the specific function of the dogs, as may fellow employees and others. Because epilepsy is not usually visible except during seizures, people may not understand the role of the dog, be afraid of him, or want to treat him as a pet instead of a working dog. While dogs for the blind are well accepted, the seizure-alert dog's role is more subtle as he accompanies someone without an obvious disability and may seem to serve no function unless there is a crisis.

However, just having the dog around can make a tremendous difference for some people, and may even improve a person's epilepsy. It is well documented that people who are enjoyably occupied have fewer seizures, and people who know they can depend on their dog feel more confident and so undertake more. The reassurance factor is by no means to be lightly dismissed given that so many people's seizures are brought on by stress or fear. With a dog, 64-year-old Betty gained the confidence to look after her 14-month-old granddaughter, something she had previously believed impossible. Dogs may also reduce stress for parents of children with epilepsy, who may be afraid to go to bed for fear their child may have a seizure, or may feel obliged to sleep in the same room in case their child needs their help during the night – something which can persist for many years, depriving a child of independence and the whole family of privacy and space.

The ketogenic diet

The ketogenic diet is a very fat-rich diet originally used as a treatment for children with difficult-to-control epilepsy, and now receiving renewed interest as a treatment still mainly for children, though there have been reports of some adults using it with success. It is often viewed rather dubiously as being fiddly, demanding and unpalatable, and with a varying success rate as regards seizure control, and with potentially unhealthy side effects. However, recent research from Johns Hopkins University in the USA, a centre for keto treatment and research, suggests that it can be both well tolerated and effective, and also that it doesn't have to be followed for ever; many children discontinue it after being seizure-free for two years. This diet is not a do-it-yourself eating plan to follow at home. It does need expert administration by a doctor trained in the ketogenic diet.

The main feature of the ketogenic diet is its high fat content, involving a food intake made up of 80–90 per cent fat such as butter, cream, oils, eggs and fat meat. For example, a typical breakfast might include eggs with several slices of bacon and hot chocolate made with 36 per cent cream. A main meal might be steak with cream sauce, lettuce with mayonnaise dressing, and a whipped cream sundae.

This extremely high fat content diet mimics the effects of fasting, described in the Bible and the Middle Ages as a way of controlling seizures. During starvation, the body first uses its store of glucose and glycogen and then begins to burn the stored body fat. When there is not enough glucose, the fats cannot be completely burned and ketone bodies (acetoacetate and beta hydroxybutyrate) are left as the residue of incompletely burned fat. It is the high level of these ketones that appear to suppress seizures – it is not known exactly how, but it is thought to affect the way the brain metabolizes ketones, which in turn affects seizure activity. Another theory is that the high fat levels help repair the myelin sheaths around the nerves of the brain.

The diet's other peculiarity is a strict limitation of carbohydrates such as bread, rice, pasta and sugar – so much so that patients may even have to monitor their toothpaste or vitamins for their sugar content or even suntan oil which may contain enough carbohydrate in the form of sorbitol to be absorbed through the skin and lower the ketone level, resulting in a seizure. Fluids are also restricted. Meals are prescribed to the last gram like medicines, carefully calculated for the individual. The died needs to be followed for up to three months before improvements can be seen.

There are drawbacks and side effects. The diet lacks essential nutrients such as vitamins B and C, and calcium, which must be given as sugar-free supplements. Side effects include higher cholesterol levels (including very high cholesterol levels, hypercholesterolemia), constipation, kidney stones, vomiting, dehydration, anaemia, loss of minerals in the bones, recurrent infections, and lethargy. However, as far as children are concerned, studies in progress suggest that only a few of them have a substantial increase in their cholesterol and triglycerides; the long-term effects of the diet on heart disease and stroke are unknown but few children remain on the diet long enough for this to happen. If properly calculated, the child should grow normally.

Originally prescribed for children with epilepsy in the 1920s in America, the diet slipped out of fashion after phenytoin was discovered in 1938 and more attention was given to new drugs in the 1950s. More recently, however, it has achieved more vogue, though its effect remains controversial and variable. Older studies suggest that an estimated third of those who tried it had seizures largely controlled, a third had substantial improvement, and a third no real benefit. More recent research from Johns Hopkins found that the diet was in general well tolerated and that after six months 31 per cent of those who tried it had over 90 per cent seizure control, 19 per cent had 50–90 per cent seizure control, and 19 per cent had under 50 per cent.

For how to get hold of more information on the ketogenic diet, ask your doctor or epilepsy specialist, or contact an epilepsy support organization, or see Further reading and Useful addresses at the end of this book.

Tomorrow's high-tech treatments

Research promises a plethora of futuristic treatments for epilepsy. Experiments have explored new forms of electronic stimulation of the brain, developed along the same lines as VNS; and other implanted devices to deliver medication directly to areas of the brain from where seizures start, which might make the drug more effective but avoid side effects to the rest of the body. Brain cell transplant is another possibility, with the idea being that transplanted immature brain cells would take on the shape and functions of damaged or missing neurons. This has been shown to happen in animal studies, and one Boston medical centre made epilepsy history by transplanting about half a million fetal pig brain cells (around the size of two drops of water) into the brain of a man with severe epilepsy.

However, without wishing to cast a damper on future possibilities, many doctors would be more than content to see epilepsy treated more effectively with the methods which already exist. The campaign 'Out of the Shadows – A Global Campaign Against Epilepsy', run by the World Health Organization (WHO), together with the International League Against Epilepsy (ILAE) and the International Bureau for Epilepsy (IBE), was launched in order to fight the under-recognition and under-treatment of epilepsy which exist worldwide. According to ILAE President, Dr Edward Reynolds, in developing countries particularly, because of ignorance, fear and stigma, epilepsy is often ignored rather than being recognized as a medical, treatable condition.

Meanwhile, much nearer home, resources in the UK for epilepsy are traditionally underfunded, with specialist centres being relatively few and far between. This said, intractable or hard-to-control epilepsy remains a major problem, and who knows which treatment of the future might be the one to improve seizure control and quality of life for people with the more difficult forms of epilepsy?

5

The hormonal factor

For a woman with epilepsy, the normal convolutions of coming to terms with her sexuality and reproductive powers may be further complicated both by her condition and its treatment. Acknowledging this is one of the important recent advances in epilepsy care. In the past decade it has become much more recognized that epilepsy can affect areas such as menstruation, contraception, fertility and menopause; and treatment is much more tailored to take into account the particular needs of women.

Horror stories abound of the bad old days when women were disbelieved when they said their seizures coincided with menstruation or when they were given no advice about how their drugs might impact on contraception, family planning or pregnancy. Pre-conception counselling especially, covered in the next chapter, is a major move forward.

Unfortunately, the murky past has still not totally gone for many women with epilepsy. A survey by the British Epilepsy Association of 2,000 women showed that women want and need more information about issues such as contraception, pregnancy, birth and the menopause. For example, the survey showed that nearly half of the women taking the contraceptive pill felt they had not been given enough information about the pill and their treatment. However, the information is available – if women are prepared to ask for it. The suggestion that women should be much more prepared to question the experts about their treatment can be seen as part of a general move by people with epilepsy in taking more responsibility for their treatment, and in having more of an active role in the management of their epilepsy.

Having a clear knowledge of how epilepsy and its treatment can impact on reproductive functions will make for greater personal and sexual confidence – or as clear a knowledge as possible. This is still an area where research is needed as doctors are not always certain about the exact links between your hormones and epilepsy. However, hormonal aspects of epilepsy are receiving more medical interest, and it is known that the two major reproductive hormones, oestrogen and progesterone, may affect epilepsy as they influence excitability in brain cells: oestrogen being excitatory (makes brain cells more likely to fire in a seizure), and progesterone inhibitory (dampens cell activity down so making a seizure less likely). Also, seizures may affect areas in the brain which regulate the production of these hormones, in particular, the hypothalamus and limbic structures, which in turn may impact on aspects of reproduction such as periods and fertility.

Seizures around menstruation (catamenial epilepsy)

Many women find they have more seizures around ovulation (which usually takes place roughly halfway through a cycle), or that their seizures cluster around menstruation, a phenomenon known as catamenial epilepsy. Some women, especially those with mixed seizure types, also show increased activity on the EEG during menstruation. Catamenial epilepsy has been known about since antiquity when, like so much else, it was attributed to the phases of the moon.

Women with partial epilepsy, especially temporal lobe epilepsy, seem to be most likely to have catamenial epilepsy. Interestingly, though, it isn't just women who have seizures in cycles; some research has shown that nearly a third of men have a cyclical increase in tonic-clonic seizures within 8–46 day cycles; and before puberty girls may have recurrent clusters of seizures each month until puberty, when the seizures become catamenial.

This is still a controversial area which is not properly understood. Several theories have been suggested to explain why the menstrual cycle should affect epilepsy, including cyclic changes in the immune system. It has also been suggested that, rather than the epilepsy itself becoming worse, women's perceptions of the epilepsy change before a period because they go into a different mood state or suffer premenstrual tension (it is worth saying that the exponents of many such theories are men!).

One of the main theories, however, is that seizures around periods may be due to fluctuations in the two major reproductive hormones, oestrogen and progesterone, which rise and fall in the menstrual cycle. The effects of those hormones on brain excitability, mentioned above, are at the root of this theory. Roughly speaking, oestrogen seems to be the 'baddy', lowering seizure threshold, while progesterone seems to offer more protection against seizures, increasing seizure threshold.

Studies have shown that, in women with catamenial epilepsy, more seizures take place at two specific times in the cycles – when levels of oestrogen are high, before ovulation, and when progesterone levels are low, before a period.

Some women with epilepsy do tend to have more periods when

ovulation does not take place (annovulatory cycles, when an ovum, or egg, is not produced) and/or irregular periods. Also, some women have more seizures during the second half of annovulatory cycles when progesterone levels are relatively low.

The hormonal process which brings about menstruation begins in the hypothalamus, an especially important part of the brain as it is the main point where neuronal and hormonal systems of the body interact. The hypothalamus acts as a vast control centre for a number of functions – not just menstruation, but also mood, sleep, weight and day/night rhythm. From the hypothalamus, electrical brain action stimulates the pituitary gland to send out chemical messengers which may result in the release of any one of several hormones such as adrenaline, sex hormones, milk-secreting hormones and others, all of which are associated with changes in the emotions.

To kick off menstruation, the hypothalamus releases gonadotropin-releasing hormone (GnRH), a process modulated by a variety of chemical messengers or neurotransmitters, and it has been suggested that it is at this stage of the proceedings that epilepsy interferes – right at the core of the brain.

Gonadotropin-releasing hormone is a powerful substance which stimulates the pituitary to produce two menstrual hormones – follicle-stimulating hormone (FSH) and luteinizing hormone (LH). FSH acts on one of the two ovaries to produce a follicle. This follicle in turn secretes increasing amounts of oestrogen up to ovulation, when LH causes the ripening follicle to burst and release the egg. This is when the level of oestrogen drops abruptly, and, under the influence of LH, there is a rise in progesterone, now secreted by the empty follicle which develops into a mass of cells called the corpus luteum. If the ovum or egg is not fertilized, the corpus luteum dissolves, oestrogen levels drop again along with progesterone, and the lining of the uterus is discarded as menstrual blood.

Extra medication in the week before menstruation in the form of an 'add-on' anti-epileptic such as clobazam is the commonest method of treating seizures around the time of menstruation. Other methods include treating catamenial epilepsy with the contraceptive pill to try and balance hormones more, an option which can work for many women although some find the side effects unacceptable, and increasing the usual dose of anti-epileptic just before a period. Some centres, especially in the USA, have tried treating catamenial epilepsy, as well as pre-menstrual syndrome (see below), with natural progesterone and other hormonal therapies.

Another theory is that seizures around menstruation are linked to pre-menstrual water retention, which upsets the normal balance of the anti-epileptic drug in your body, so making it less effective. For this reason, doctors have commonly treated catamenial epilepsy with diuretics to reduce fluid, though this seems to be falling out of favour as it quite often doesn't work.

You may find that simple self-help measures, including attention to diet and exercise, will help you feel better around periods, and these are outlined below.

Pre-menstrual tension

An estimated 40 per cent of all women are believed to suffer pre-menstrual tension (PMT – known in the US as pre-menstrual syndrome, or PMS), and women with epilepsy generally seem much the same, as around 43 per cent of them report it, but this figure goes up to 75 per cent in women with catamenial seizures, who may have severe PMT. PMT is marked by symptoms such as depression, fatigue, irritability, migraine, bloating or water retention, sleep problems and food cravings, which tend to appear regularly at set times each month, perhaps five days or so before a period (remember the role of the hypothalamus as a control centre for many of these functions). It has been suggested that PMT is due to high levels of oestrogen and low levels of progesterone at this phase in the menstrual cycle, although not all researchers agree. The onset of PMT seems to follow some shock to the endocrine system such as menarche (first menstruation), childbirth, hysterectomy, going on or off a birth-control pill, or major life stress. PMT seems to be hereditary and symptoms can become worse with age.

Links between severe PMT and epilepsy are currently under research by some American neurologists (Dietrich Blumer, an expert on epilepsy and mood disorder, and colleagues at the Baptist Memorial Hospital, Tennessee) who have found that the symptoms of severe PMT are identical to the symptoms of an epileptic phenomenon known as 'interictal dysphoric disorder'. Symptoms of both disorders are said to include extreme mood swings, anxiety, a lack of energy, insomnia or hypersomnia, and pain, appearing in an intermittent pattern, together with heightened irritability and sometimes explosive rage. The researchers note that there is a high incidence of severe PMT among women with epilepsy, and that women diagnosed with interictal dysphoric disorder find it is often much worse just before their periods begin. Interictal dysphoric disorder is treated with anticonvulsants and antidepressants, a regimen that Blumer et al. have now used success-fully to treat PMT in women both with and without epilepsy. This area continues to be researched.

There is no doubt that severe PMT can make life a misery – and this means not just the four or five days before a period, but sometimes the first two or three days of a period as well. However, some women have found simple self-help measures quite effective.

Coping with PMT

- Keep a note of symptoms to help you decide whether or not you do suffer from PMT and, if so, at which times of the month you need to take action. Typically PMT symptoms appear five days before your period starts.
- Discuss any symptoms you do find with your doctor, family and friends.
- Don't be put off by people saying 'It's all in your head' – it's a biochemical disorder, not a psychological one.
- Eat six small meals a day or three smallish meals plus snacks to help keep blood sugar levels steady. You should eat regularly throughout your cycle but this may be particularly important after ovulation when changes in hormone levels alter your biochemistry, making you more susceptible to low blood sugar reactions, such as irritability, migraine, panic, tears and angry outbursts (see advice on healthy eating in Chapter 7).
- Exercise regularly, if possible three times a week all month.
- Cut down on salt. Since salt holds water, reducing salt intake may help reduce bloating and water retention.
- Be sure to drink plenty of water – drinking a lot will not make water retention worse. Some evidence suggests that eating starchy food every three hours may help water retention, such as toast, a biscuit, or some pasta. Other people have found that eating more protein helps, or potassium-rich foods such as bananas, tomato juice, or orange juice.
- The B vitamins, especially B6, are sometimes used to reduce bloating and depression, and they seem to help control carbohydrate cravings. As taking one B vitamin increases your need for the others, you should take this as a B-complex, not in isolation.
- Reduce stress if possible. Take things easy just before your period. Set aside some time to nap, listen to music, read, or go for a walk. Being alone can be very important to some women at this time.

- Be wary of evening primrose oil, often recommended for PMT. There have been reports of it causing seizures, especially in those with temporal lobe epilepsy.

Contraception – the pill

I can't take the pill because it's affected by my medication. This I had to find out for myself because neither my GP nor my family planning clinic knew about it.
Julie

I don't take the pill but epilepsy has not affected my choice of contraception. My family planning clinic were very well informed about contraception for women with epilepsy.
Anthea

It does still happen that women with epilepsy are not told about the effects of anti-epileptic drugs on the contraceptive pill either by their regular doctor or their family planning clinic – according to the British Epilepsy Association survey mentioned at the opening of this chapter, only half of those surveyed had received advice about the possible effects of anti-epileptic drugs on contraception. This can lead to litigation – there have been cases of women becoming pregnant and suing doctors on the grounds that they had not been advised of the possible failure of contraception.

The problem relates to low-dose forms of the contraceptive pill (30 microgrammes oestrogen), as certain anti-epileptic drugs speed up the way the liver breaks down the pill, and can to a certain degree 'cancel out' its effect. The drugs which make the pill less effective are 'enzyme inducers' and include phenobarbitone, primidone, phenytoin, carbama-zepine, topiramate and oxcarbazepine (a drug due to be licensed which may affect the pill). The low-dose pill is as effective as usual if you are taking sodium valproate, vigabatrin, clobazam, lamotrigine, gabapentin, ethosuximide and piracetam.

This is a particularly sensitive issue because of the implications of an unplanned pregnancy. Certain drugs can sometimes cause defects in a developing baby (see next chapter). To be on the safe side, if you are taking an enzyme-inducing drug, it's been recommended that you start on a pill with 50 microgrammes of oestrogen, though this is something to discuss with your doctor. Any breakthrough bleeding between periods is likely to be a sign that the dose of oestrogen is not high enough. If this does happen, use other precautions and consult your doctor, who will probably raise the oestrogen dose. However, even a higher-dose pill is less effective (as regards contraception) than if enzyme-inducing drugs are not taken – about as effective as barrier methods. So, if preventing pregnancy is essential, it may be wise to consider using additional contraception as well, such as the condom or cap.

If you are planning to become pregnant in the not-too-distant future, another option could be to think ahead and consider changing drugs. Carbamazepine, sodium valproate, phenytoin and primidone may affect an unborn baby, so it may be suggested that you switch anyway several months before planning to conceive (see next chapter for more detail). Of course, if you are relatively happy and settled on your current drug, you may feel this is an unnecessary upheaval, but it could be something to bear in mind for the future.

One potential advantage of the pill is that, because it regulates hormones, it may result in better seizure control. However, the pill is not for everyone, and many women make contraceptive choices quite unconnected with epilepsy. Some women with epilepsy feel that, being on one set of drugs, they don't want to have to take the pill too, either because of side effects (in some women, the side effects of the pill can be similar to those for some anti-epileptic drugs), or because of the inconvenience of having to remember to take it, especially if they suffer from a poor memory.

General health reasons, as with all women, may be an important consideration. The benefits of the pill include convenience, shorter, more regular periods, and increased protection against ovarian cysts, ovarian and endometrial (lining of the uterus) cancer, non-cancerous breast tumours, pelvic inflammatory disease, and anaemia. The disadvantages include irregular bleeding for the first few months, increased appetite, depression or moodiness, headaches and/or dizziness, nausea and vomiting, scant or missed periods, weight change, high blood pressure, and breast tenderness. Serious problems related to use of the pill are very rare, though the chances of developing blood clots, heart attack, high blood pressure, stroke, or liver tumours are slightly greater in women who take it. The risk is increased if you have a history of previous blood vessel disorders, have high blood pressure or high cholesterol levels, have diabetes, or suffer from migraine. Smokers, those who are very overweight, and women over 35 are also at higher risk.

One further small proviso – while women with epilepsy may use any form of contraception going, if you choose to have an IUD (intra uterine device or coil) fitted, there is a very small risk of having a seizure when it is inserted. Make sure the person fitting the device knows you have epilepsy.

Fertility

One in six couples in the general population have difficulty conceiving a baby. Some studies have suggested that fertility may be slightly reduced in women with epilepsy. For example, one study by London doctors, reported in the *Lancet*, found that fertility rates among women in the general population were 33 per cent higher than among women with epilepsy. But, other studies have questioned this – a four-year study from Iceland and Columbia University, New York, found that there was no evidence of altered fertility among people with epilepsy unless they had mental retardation or cerebral palsy. The study, of more than 200 women, found that they had the same number of children as people without epilepsy – two.

Some women do find it difficult to get pregnant. The reason is that, as described in the section on menstruation, seizures can upset the hormones associated with fertility. If you cannot get pregnant after a year of trying you should discuss it with your doctor, especially if you have irregular periods, as polycystic ovary syndrome (see below) is a possibility and can be treated. If your doctor refers you to an infertility treatment clinic, you should have no problems with the hormone-based fertility drugs such as clomiphene, though a few women experience a very small rise in seizures. However, you will probably find it best to complete any other drug changes first.

There have been recent reports that therapy with sodium valproate beginning in childhood/adolescence may predispose towards the polycystic ovary syndrome, a possible cause of infertility. Studies have shown that changing to lamotrigine is likely to reverse these changes.

Maximizing your chances of pregnancy

There are various self-help measures you and your partner can take to boost fertility and encourage a pregnancy:

- Lose weight if you are overweight; alternatively, gain weight if you are too thin. Extremes of weight can impact on reproductive hormones and decrease fertility.

- Give up smoking.
- Cut out alcohol.
- Eat a healthy diet as suggested in Chapter 7.
- Try and minimize environmental hazards at work or elsewhere such as lead, cadmium, mercury, ethylene oxide, vinyl chloride, radioactivity and x-rays.
- All the above can benefit men as well as women. Male fertility can also be affected by prescription drugs for ulcers or psoriasis, and warm temperatures which can affect the genitals, such as over-hot baths. There have been a few case reports of high dose sodium valproate therapy producing reversible infertility in men.
- Try to make love when you're ovulating, but without it becoming a chore. Regular periods usually suggest that ovulation is taking place. Otherwise, signs that you are ovulating include pain on ovulation (*mittelschmerz*) on one side or other of the abdomen, which can be quite severe for a day or two; and changes in vaginal mucus, which typically becomes thicker. Home testing kits, based on detecting a hormone in the urine, can also pinpoint when you're ovulating.

Polycystic ovary syndrome

There has been a lot of concern recently about sodium valproate taken during childhood later causing polycystic ovaries. Polycystic ovary syndrome (PCOS) is one of the most common causes of infertility in women and may also impact on overall as well as reproductive health.

Thought to affect around 6 per cent of all women, it seems to be more common in women with epilepsy who are taking sodium valproate. In two Finnish studies, 50–60 per cent of women treated with sodium valproate before the age of 20 had polycystic ovaries. The most common symptom is irregular or infrequent periods; other signs include prominent facial or body hair, severe acne, thinning hair on the head, and obesity.

The disease gets its name from many small cysts which build up inside the ovaries due to abnormal hormone levels.

Self-help measures which have benefited some women include eating a healthy diet, in particular a high-protein diet excluding sugar, keeping weight down and exercising anyway will help boost general and reproductive health.

As regards treatment, obviously if you take sodium valproate, you and your doctor will probably want to consider a change of drug –

again, this applies particularly if you are planning a pregnancy, as sodium valproate is a drug whose use is not recommended in pregnancy. Other treatments for polycystic ovaries include use of the contraceptive pill to lower androgen levels and establish regular menstruation, sometimes in combination with other drugs, and surgery.

Menopause

It might seem logical that the same hormonal variables which affect women's epilepsy around menstruation would also have an impact on menopause, but this is an area where there is very little research.

The effect of menopause on seizures seems partly to depend on whether they are catamenial; women with catamenial epilepsy do sometimes find that their seizures improve or disappear after menopause. But, other women find that seizures increase. Rarely, seizures may start for the first time around this time of life, though the reason why is again not always clear. In most women, it just seems to happen. As epilepsy can develop at any stage of life, some women may develop epilepsy at this time coincidentally but it does seem to happen slightly more commonly than might be expected by chance. There is an increasing incidence of epilepsy as women get older but it is most likely related to the fact that the incidence of cerebrovascular disease increases with age.

HRT and epilepsy

HRT and epilepsy is another area where there is very little research, but, in general, women with epilepsy are advised to try HRT with the proviso that some will experience an increase in seizures, in which case they should inform their doctor; some will also find the side effects untenable. HRT is commonly prescribed at menopause to relieve unpleasant oestrogen withdrawal symptoms such as hot flushes, mood changes, irritability, depression, sweating and insomnia.

HRT is also commonly prescribed to prevent and treat osteoporosis, or bone-thinning. Changes in oestrogen at the menopause mean a woman starts losing the protection offered by this hormone and becomes exposed to changes in the way calcium is metabolized. Also, some epilepsy drugs contribute to bone-thinning; enzyme-inducing anticonvulsants, such as phenobarbitone, primidone, phenytoin and carbamazepine speed up the metabolism of vitamin D. Vitamin D is needed for the body to be able to absorb calcium, so this can have profound effects on calcium loss. Women who are taking these drugs are most at risk of osteoporosis and most in need of trying HRT.

Doctors do not universally agree about how long HRT should be given, and in what form. Oestrogen may be used on its own, but, because of the known effect of oestrogen on seizures, epilepsy specialists strongly recommend that HRT is given mixed with progesterone to help balance the oestrogen. Sometimes a small amount of testosterone may be added, particularly for women who have lost their libido, and calcium and vitamin D supplements can be recommended too. While oestrogen may in theory make seizures more likely, the small doses used in HRT do not usually cause any problems. However, some women even with an oestrogen-progesterone HRT combination, have a rise in seizures on HRT and so may have to abandon treatment.

Some women are also concerned about other side effects of HRT – some find they cannot tolerate it because of side effects, while others are concerned about possible long-term effects such as cancer. On the other hand, there is a small amount of evidence that HRT helps protect you against heart disease because of the protective effect of oestrogen, and that survival for women with breast cancer is greatly increased if they have taken HRT.

There is increasing interest in natural methods of dealing with the menopause which avoid HRT altogether and you may want to try healthy living measures which may cut down on or eliminate your need for HRT (see Further reading).

Preventing osteoporosis – take action now

Because anti-epileptic drugs affect the way calcium is metabolized by the body, women with epilepsy are advised to think about their long-term bone health from the word go. Women in general, who have a one-in-three chance of developing osteoporosis (thinning bones) in later life, are advised not to wait until their fifties but to start taking action in their thirties when the skeleton is still forming. For the woman with epilepsy, though, this could be a concern which starts with drug treatment.

Osteoporosis in the UK affects 3 million and causes more than 200,000 fractures a year, around 40 of which a day prove fatal. If you're concerned, you could contact the National Osteoporosis Society for further advice; and a bone density scan is available on the NHS to all at high risk of osteoporosis.

Meanwhile, healthy habits to carry you through into old age include looking after your diet, exercise, and menstrual health, as well as avoiding dangers.

- **Diet.** Apart from following general healthy eating guidelines (see Chapter 7), the key nutrient is calcium, which builds and maintains bones. The best sources are dairy products such as milk, cheese and yoghurt – low-fat varieties generally contain as much calcium as full-fat ones. Other good sources are bony fish such as sardines, tofu, watercress, nuts, seeds, carbonated water, baked beans, and dried fruit such as figs. Calcium supplements are also available, but discuss this with your doctor first – on the whole, calcium is best absorbed with food, and as part of a varied, balanced diet. You also need vitamin D to help you absorb calcium; around 80 per cent of our intake comes from daylight, but it is also found in full-fat dairy products, fortified cereals, margarine and low-fat spreads, oily fish such as salmon, tuna and fish liver oil, and eggs.

- **The right exercise.** Bones stay strong by being used. Weight-bearing exercise is best, which means anything which loads bones, such as aerobics, dancing, jogging, ball sports, and brisk walking. Studies show a significant difference between those who took little exercise and those who walked seven miles a week – that's half an hour a day outdoor exercise. Don't overdo it, as very intensive training may weaken bones, especially if you're not eating enough – athletes and dancers are at high risk of osteoporosis.

- **Periods.** Anything which impairs periods needs attention because the sex hormones are the most important factor in osteoporosis, and if you diet to excess you can lose your periods. This can apply to normally 'slim' women as well as women with anorexia if periods are light or missed. However, this can be more difficult for women with epilepsy who are more prone to irregular periods. Make sure you eat a healthy, regular diet, and again consult your doctor for further help.

- **Avoid dangers.** Dangers include common health enemies such as smoking, too much alcohol and too much caffeine from tea, coffee and cola, which can all deplete bone density. Fizzy drinks are high in phosphorous, which can upset the body's calcium balance. Laxatives and bran fibre can increase your loss of calcium and other nutrients. Finally, stress, as well as triggering seizures, can also be bad for bones as it causes the release of adrenaline into the body, and too much adrenaline has a harmful dissolving effect on bone.

6

Having a baby

Most women with epilepsy have perfectly normal pregnancies and deliveries, which is just as well as, traditionally, many of them have been allowed to go through their pregnancies without a word of counselling from their medical carers with regard to managing their epilepsy during pregnancy, particularly with regard to anti-epileptic drugs. Even today, a recent survey by the British Epilepsy Association of 2,000 women showed that over a third of women who had children said they had received no advice at all during pregnancy, while only a quarter had discussed the issues with a doctor before conception. Only 10 per cent could remember being told that anticonvulsants pose a danger to the unborn baby.

However, with today's greater awareness of the special needs of women with epilepsy, your doctor should be able to advise you on pre-conception care and pregnancy. The majority of drugs for epilepsy can pose risks, and proper prescribing may reduce these dangers. If your own doctor cannot help, then another doctor may be able to. This may mean seeking a second opinion, though not all GPs undertake obstetric care, so it may be worth checking with your surgery whether you should consult another doctor for pregnancy and childbirth anyway. You should also ask your GP for referral if you have access to a local epilepsy specialist running a pre-conception clinic. But, no matter whom you do consult, the vital point is that you do it well in advance of becoming pregnant – ideally six months to one year before conception if possible.

This is because the prospect of pregnancy raises a number of questions which may take several months to tackle. How easy will it be for me to become pregnant? Should I come off my drugs? Above all, will my baby be all right? All women worry about this at some point during their pregnancy, but it may have more relevance for women with epilepsy because of the risk of drugs affecting the baby, which is why it is so important to be informed before becoming pregnant, and to ensure as far as possible that you are happy and relaxed with your medical care.

The risks are discussed in more detail below, but broadly, most women in the general population have a 97–98 per cent chance of giving birth to a healthy baby; for women on anti-epileptic drugs, the risks are slightly higher but they still have around a 94–96 per cent chance or more of having a healthy baby. Problems tend to be mainly minor ones, and the risks can be reduced or avoided by changes in drugs. Worry about the baby needs to be kept in proportion, especially during pregnancy itself, a notoriously sensitive time of surging hormones, emotional swings and physical challenges which can be tiring and stressful even for the healthiest of mothers. Being informed about the risks – which are small – should not mean being over-anxious about them. **With proper planning, most complications can be reduced.**

Pre-conception care

Planning a pregnancy is vital for anyone, but even more so for women with epilepsy. Ideally, you should have been counselled in detail about this from childhood or early adolescence, although in real life you usually tend to find out as you go along! However much or little you know, as already stated, the most important point is to try and have counselling before becoming pregnant if possible. The unborn baby is most vulnerable during the first 12 weeks of pregnancy when all the major organs are developing, so that any adjustments to drug treatment should be made before becoming pregnant.

Having said that, it is still by no means uncommon for women to turn up at the doctor's two or three months pregnant and still taking anti-epileptic drugs which pose a risk to the developing baby. But, whatever you do, don't panic and suddenly stop taking your anti-epileptic drugs, as this can precipitate a lot of seizures which can be serious for you and possibly the baby. Remember, the vast majority of women with epilepsy do have perfectly normal babies. See your doctor, start taking folic acid, and make sure you have antenatal screening – ultrasound scans and other tests can provide reassurance that your baby is developing normally (see Tests and checks during pregnancy, below).

Ideally a team of three doctors – your GP, epilepsy specialist and obstetrician – should be involved in your pregnancy, so it may take time and several visits to cover all the points, especially if you are considering changing or withdrawing drugs, a process which will need medical monitoring. Make a list of points to discuss if you feel you may otherwise forget them. Points which may be considered include:

- taking a medical history which thoroughly reappraises your epilepsy as well as your general and sexual health;

- how soon you want to become pregnant;
- any fertility problems;
- how effective your contraception is now;
- if you are still having seizures;
- lifestyle questions or other concerns;
- folic acid supplementation;
- genetic counselling;
- withdrawing from or changing drugs.

The rest of this section looks at these points in more detail.

Medical history

Pregnancy presents an ideal time for reassessing your epilepsy completely, especially if first time round you were diagnosed just on the basis of medical history and EEG. Now is a good time to have specialist reappraisal and brain scans, especially MRI. This re-investigation can serve many purposes – to check for any lesions or scars within the brain, to make sure that you are on the right drugs, or to see if indeed you still need treatment at all.

One particular reason for re-investigating your epilepsy is to check whether your epilepsy is lesional, that is, whether it stems from scarring or damage to brain tissue, and this can be detected by MRI. Blood flow increases by 30 per cent during pregnancy, and this can put extra pressure on previously unsuspected conditions such as malformations in the veins of the brain, or aneurysms (when blood vessel walls are stretched by extra pressure of blood), or, rarely, tumour. Such conditions, which might otherwise complicate a pregnancy, may effectively be dealt with by surgery before a pregnancy begins. In one study of pre-conception counselling, 9 per cent of the women had a previously undetected lesion. The main (but very rare) risk is that the extra blood flow could put pressure on delicate areas which, if they rupture, can result in haemorrhage, depriving the unborn baby of oxygen, potentially making your epilepsy worse, and in extreme cases even putting your own life at risk. Again, these risks have to be kept in perspective but it is worth having them checked if you can.

Women with epilepsy are automatically considered to be high-risk pregnancies, but your doctor will also need to assess any other potential risk factors such as age (i.e., if you're very young or over 35), problems with a past pregnancy, or other health conditions such as asthma, diabetes, heart problems, or high blood pressure or hypertension.

Fertility problems

Pre-conception counselling offers the chance to mention any worries you have about becoming pregnant. In particular, you should mention irregular periods, which can indicate you're not ovulating regularly and so may have fewer chances of becoming pregnant. Your doctor can check your ovaries to make sure you do not have polycystic ovaries (see Chapter 5) and refer you to a fertility clinic if necessary.

How soon you want to become pregnant

Because of careers, many women delay pregnancy until their late 30s and then feel under pressure from the biological timeclock and want to start a family as soon as possible. If the epilepsy is well controlled and you are on a relatively low dose of a drug which does not seem to be teratogenic (i.e., likely to cause defects in the baby), there is probably no reason why you should wait an undue time, though you should consider taking a folic acid supplement beforehand (see Folic acid supplementation, below).

There can be reasons for delaying pregnancy. Sometimes, women prefer to postpone pregnancy in the hopes of achieving better control of their epilepsy, through drug changes, which can take several months, perhaps in combination with lifestyle measures such as better diet and more sleep.

How effective your contraception is now

Because drug changes take time, to be caught by an unexpected pregnancy halfway through a drug change is not ideal. So, you may need to change or reinforce contraception, for example by your partner using barrier methods in addition to your current contraception.

Withdrawing from or changing drugs

The consultant told us that the results of my brain scan showed there were still abnormalities in my brain and that if I stopped taking my drugs I would almost certainly have seizures again. But, if I wanted a baby, he felt that it would be best for me to come off the drugs as there was a chance they could cause deformities in the baby. The consultant said it was unlikely the seizures would harm the baby. I felt that the seizures were terrible, but not as terrible as going through life childless. My drug dose was reduced immediately and I was weaned off gradually. The next six months dragged, as we

couldn't start trying for a baby until my system was clear of the drugs. But, once given the all-clear, to my delight I fell pregnant straight away. Sure enough, seizures continued throughout pregnancy, but, after a very worrying time, I gave birth to a perfect little girl, Amelia.
Julie

If you're settled on one drug and able to lead a normal life with minimal side effects, the prospect of changing or abandoning drugs can be somewhat daunting. On the other hand, taking drugs which might affect the baby is a very worrying question for many women, and the question of whether they can withdraw from their medication will naturally be uppermost in the minds of many. Indeed, many women don't take or reduce their drugs while pregnant through fear of the effect on the baby.

Generally, the risks seem highest with certain older drugs such as sodium valproate, carbamazepine, phenytoin, primidone and phenobarbitone. The risks seem to be highest with phenytoin (cleft palate and hare lip and heart abnormalities) and sodium valproate (malformation of the fingers and penis and spina bifida). Carbamazepine can possibly cause spina bifida and may sometimes be associated with low birth weight and slow initial development. Topiramate, one of the new drugs, may also cause abnormalities as animal studies suggest it causes deformities of the arms and legs. But, other new anti-epileptic drugs, gabapentin and lamotrigine, do not seem to cause damage in animals though they have not been in use long enough to be completely sure that no damage would be caused to human babies. Some doctors believe that these two drugs will become the drugs of choice for women with epilepsy who wish to become pregnant, depending on the type of epilepsy they have. Vigabatrin is also probably safer than the older drugs. Risks for some drugs are dose-related – i.e. they are reduced if the dose of the medication is lower.

While everyone's circumstances are different, average risk potential can be roughly estimated as follows. Women who have had seizures but are currently not having seizures or taking anti-epileptic drugs have approximately a 3 per cent risk of problems. Women whose epilepsy is controlled by one drug have around a 4 per cent chance of problems. Women with uncontrolled epilepsy who are taking more than one drug have a higher risk of problems, perhaps 6–10 per cent. A father's epilepsy, controlled or not, seems to have no effect on the baby's development.

Defects which do occur are mostly minor, like small nails. The most common more serious abnormality is cleft lip or palate, which accounts for about a third of abnormalities, and which is easily corrected by operation after the birth. Other defects include malformation of the face such as eyes set too far apart (hypertelorism), and malformation of the fingers such as webbed fingers (syndactyly). Other possible complications include malformation of the penis (hypospadias) and reduced birth weight with initial slow development, though many children do seem to fight through this.

> Maria was born with slight congenital heart defects, and low birth weight (she weighed just 4 lbs/2 kilos) after her mother, not warned of the risks of anti-epileptic drugs, had continued taking phenytoin throughout pregnancy. During her first two years of life, things did not look promising: Maria was frequently very ill, and was much slower than normal in gaining developmental milestones such as sitting and walking. However, in her third year she suddenly started going from strength to strength and now, aged seven, is a normal healthy little girl.

Much more rarely, problems will be more serious – heart abnormalities such as a hole in the heart, and neural tube defects such as spina bifida, when the spinal cord fails to develop normally. The risk of neural tube defects in the general population is 0.2–0.5 per cent. Sodium valproate during pregnancy bears a 2–3 per cent risk of neural tube defects, and carbamazepine a 1 per cent risk. Sometimes, it may be possible that some of the risk relates to genetic predisposition, so it may be worth checking your family medical history to see if any of these conditions have existed in other members.

There have been reports of women with epilepsy taking legal action against various health authorities after giving birth to children with abnormalities linked to anticonvulsant drugs, mostly sodium valproate. The birth defects include spina bifida and foetal valproate syndrome, marked by a wide-bridged nose, wide forehead, mental retardation, and difficulties with movement. The women say they were never warned about the effect drugs could have on their baby, even though the risks of sodium valproate are well known.

Withdrawing from drugs altogether, which your doctor may consider after two to three seizure-free years, needs careful consideration for health and other reasons such as driving and employment. Drug withdrawal does need medical supervision because of the potentially life-threatening risk of prolonged seizure, or status epilepticus.

The risks of seizures to an unborn baby are generally considered to be relatively small. Occasionally, in a prolonged seizure late in pregnancy, a baby's heart can slow slightly, but this rarely causes serious consequences.

If you don't feel confident about total withdrawal, or if your doctor feels it is not possible, or you are still having seizures, another option is lowering the dose so that you are on the lowest possible effective dose. Women on a combination of drugs may also want to consider going down to one drug, using the most appropriate drug.

It may seem strange, but, if you stay on your medication, you may find that the dose has to be increased as pregnancy progresses. This is because several factors affect how well your body processes drugs in pregnancy. Your body uses up more medication than usual because of the 'diluting' effect of the extra blood, water and weight which is gained. Other metabolic changes may affect drug metabolism, especially changes in the liver which speed up the destruction of many anti-epileptic drugs.

Finally, another possible way to gain control before pregnancy is surgery. As already discussed in Chapter 4, this isn't used routinely, but could certainly be an option depending on the results of MRI. One point to bear in mind is that this will almost certainly delay pregnancy for a year or two or even longer while all the relevant tests are made, and, if in the end it's decided yours is not a suitable case for surgery, you may then have to face more delay while drug treatment is sorted out.

Lifestyle questions or other concerns

These may be concerns specific to epilepsy or more general matters. It is surprisingly common for women (with epilepsy or without it) to have a particular worry about something which may have happened in early pregnancy, such as having had a few drinks or having done a strenuous work-out at the gym. Your doctor can provide reassurance that the vast majority of unborn babies are quite tough and usually emerge unscathed. This can also be a chance to discuss other concerns such as the prospect of parenthood, antenatal classes, and your partner's views.

Folic acid supplementation

All women are advised to take folic acid to try and prevent neural tube defects in the baby such as spina bifida. The normal recommendation is 0.5 mg a day while trying for a baby, and for the first three months of pregnancy. Women with epilepsy are usually advised to take a much higher dose than this – 5 mg per day while trying to become pregnant or for at least one month before conception, and throughout the first three months of pregnancy. Not all doctors agree that the higher dose is necessary on the grounds that it is only *assumed* on good evidence it will prevent spina bifida due to anticonvulsants, and is not medically proven that it will, but most women would probably feel safer taking no chances. Folic acid is available in both doses over the counter at your pharmacist.

Genetic counselling

Caroline grew up believing that having epilepsy meant she wouldn't be able to have children, after a few chance remarks from her great-grandmother. She never discussed this with her mother, who could have reassured her, and it wasn't until she had her first serious boyfriend, at the age of 19, that her better-informed GP put her right during a discussion about contraception. However, when Caroline became pregnant at 27, she didn't feel entirely comfortable until after a session with a genetic counsellor, which finally reassured her that her baby had only a slightly higher chance of having epilepsy than any baby.

Some women may still grow up believing that epilepsy cuts out the chance of a family of their own. This goes back to an ancient belief that all epilepsy is inherited – which may in turn be linked to equally old superstitions about epilepsy being contagious.

Most women with epilepsy have a slightly higher chance of their baby having epilepsy compared to the rest of the population – about 1 per cent. Epilepsy is rarely inherited, though a predisposition to epilepsy may be passed on. Seizure threshold is part of a person's genetic make up, and may be passed on to children, so to some extent everyone with epilepsy has a genetic element to their condition, but this is very variable. A few types of epilepsy carry a small risk of future children inheriting epilepsy; for example, if pre-conception screening has picked up tuberous sclerosis, a genetic condition which causes epilepsy, there is a 50 to one chance of it being passed on to children.

There are some other rare types of epilepsy which can run in families. If more than one member of your family has epilepsy, it is worth telling your GP about the possibility of the epilepsy being genetic in origin.

Depending on your type of epilepsy and family history, you and your doctor may want to consider genetic counselling, which, while it won't make hard and fast predictions, can help you work out the likelihood of your baby inheriting epilepsy. So, when preparing for your doctor's appointment, it would be helpful to gather together as much information about your family medical history as possible.

Getting the attention you need

In a recent survey by the British Epilepsy Association, it was found that many women don't get the medical attention they require simply because they don't speak out. The survey found that one quarter of the women had not discussed their pregnancy with anyone. It is true that pre-conception care is a relatively recent advance in epilepsy treatment, and some older family doctors may not be fully aware of its implications. However, information and advice *is* available – from a second opinion, a specialist or a support group.

- Make a list of points to discuss with your doctor as suggested above.
- Ask specifically for referral to an epilepsy specialist if you have not already seen one. Epilepsy organizations may be able to suggest local specialist centres.
- If your own doctor cannot help, seek a second opinion. You should inform your current GP that you are doing this.
- Contact an epilepsy organization such as the British Epilepsy Association or the National Society for Epilepsy for further advice and support.
- At your 'booking in' visit or your first antenatal visit you will need to inform your midwife that you have epilepsy. It is a good idea to explain what your seizures are like – their nature, length, any pattern to them, and how often they happen. Other points to mention are your medication and whether your partner has epilepsy.

Preparing for pregnancy – what you can do

Apart from seeing your doctor and discussing and implementing any drug changes, there are some measures you can take before and during pregnancy to ensure you are in optimal health.

- Eat folate-rich foods such as fruit, vegetables such as broccoli, nuts (unless allergic), cereals, pulses, yeast extract.

- Follow the other healthy eating guidelines in Chapter 7.
- Cut out alcohol or keep it to an absolute minimum.
- Cut out smoking.
- Try and sleep more regularly. This is a particularly effective self-help measure to cut down on the possibility of seizures, but don't let it become an obsession!

Safety

Many women worry about safety during pregnancy, but usually a few commonsense precautions can minimize risks and anxieties. Falling rarely injures an unborn baby, who is snugly cushioned within the amniotic fluid.

- If possible, take a bath or shower when someone else is in the house.
- Your midwife may be able to advise on general safety issues such as safety pillows, hazards from slippery mats and trailing electrical flexes, the need for fire guards, and safety locks on bathroom doors. If you don't already have these, you may well want them once your baby becomes mobile!

When epilepsy starts during pregnancy

Some women develop epilepsy for the first time during pregnancy. The most likely cause, especially late in pregnancy, is a complication of pregnancy, pre-eclamptic toxaemia, which can result from hypertension or high blood pressure. Bedrest is traditionally prescribed for high blood pressure along with hospital monitoring, though there is no evidence that this controls high blood pressure. The only real cure is delivery, so that if near term you may be induced or given a caesarean. Magnesium salts may also be used to control seizures.

A few women appear to have seizures only while pregnant, but this is rare, and in fact it is thought that these women have had unrecognized partial (usually simple) seizures in the past, which then become secondarily generalized in pregnancy. However, seizures should always be investigated because there may be underlying causes.

Seizures during pregnancy

Many women will not notice any change in their seizure pattern during pregnancy, and some will find that control is much better. This may be related to hormonal factors, as women with catamenial epilepsy in

81

particular (epilepsy around the time of menstruation) often notice improvement, or it could just be that women are more careful about diet and rest.

Around 25–30 per cent of women will have an increase in seizure frequency, often noted between weeks 8–24, thought to be due to a number of factors including changes in the way the body metabolizes drugs in pregnancy, weight gain, sleep deprivation and pregnancy nausea.

There are ways you can maximize control:

- **Take medication regularly.** Ideally, pre-conception counselling should mean you're on the minimum dose of a relatively safe drug, but if you're not happy, see your doctor rather than just giving up your drugs altogether.

- **Sleep well.** Just when you'd think nature would arrange for you to sleep better, pregnancy often brings its own sleep complications, especially towards the end when your increased bulk can make it difficult to find a comfortable sleeping position. Overheating and pressure on the bladder can also wake you more frequently. Try catching up with naps during the day; make sure you have enough supporting pillows and not too many covers, and look at the section on relaxation in Chapter 8.

- **Pregnancy nausea and vomiting in the first 12 weeks** may mean you lose your drugs before your system has had time to absorb them. Ask your doctor for advice, as you may need to change the time you take your medication. Meanwhile, try the following tips:
  - One reason for nausea is thought to be low blood sugar (also implicated in seizures) so try starting the day with a small snack such as plain biscuits and a weak cup of tea 20 minutes before you get up.
  - Try a diet including regular small amounts of carbohydrate such as pasta, potatoes and rice, along with lots of fresh vegetables and fruit.
  - Aim to eat several small snacks a day rather than a few bigger meals.
  - Avoid fried, fatty or spicy foods.
  - Some research has shown that lack of vitamin B can cause nausea, but consult your doctor before self-supplementing, or eat foods rich in B vitamins such as meat, wholegrain products, egg yolks, fish, nuts, beans, tofu, cheese, brewer's yeast and yoghurt.

– Ginger is a traditional remedy – ginger tea from grated root or half a teaspoon of powder plus a teaspoon of honey; or crystallized ginger to nibble on.

- **Constipation** may occasionally be a factor as some people report having more seizures when constipated, and pregnancy hormones do slow down your digestive processes, making constipation more likely. Drink plenty of water, eat lots of fresh fruit and vegetables, and have some regular, gentle exercise such as walking or swimming.

Tests and checks during pregnancy

Make sure your obstetrician and midwife are aware you have epilepsy as, although you will have a named midwife, you will not always see the same person for antenatal care. You will probably have more scans than the routine number, but, basically, the main tests and checks in pregnancy are as follows.

Screening tests

These checks will give you a likely risk of having a baby with an abnormality and are non-invasive but not always completely accurate. It helps to discuss the implications with your midwife or doctor before having them, as one test tends to lead to another.

- **Ultrasound scan.** The first is done at 10–14 weeks as a dating scan, though skilled operators may provide reassuring detail about your baby's development, and the second at 18–20 weeks looks for neural tube defects. However, often only an anomalies screen at 18 weeks is offered. Some centres offer a scan at 28–30 weeks to check on the baby's growth and development. The accuracy is 70–80 per cent.

- **Nuchal fold scan.** This measures the nuchal fold at the back of the unborn baby's neck by ultrasound to look for thickening which can indicate Down's syndrome or a major malformation. It is done at 10–14 weeks and has an 80–90 per cent accuracy rate. There is no increased risk of Down's syndrome in epilepsy.

- **Triple test.** This measures hormone levels to detect Down's and neural tube defects. Done at 15–22 weeks, it has a nearly 60 per cent accuracy rate.

- **Alpha-Fetoprotein (AFP).** This is a blood test which can test for

Down's and neural tube defects. Done at 16–18 weeks, it has a nearly 80 per cent accuracy rate and is usually combined with other tests.

- **The Triple Test Plus** or **Biomark.** This also tests for Down's and neural tube defects and is available privately.

Diagnostic tests

Unlike screening tests, these give a yes or no answer and require some thought before being taken.

- **Chorionic villus sampling (CVS)** at 10–12 weeks can detect Down's, chromosomal disorders and other inherited conditions but not neural tube defects. Using ultrasound for guidance, a needle is inserted into the abdomen and a tiny sample of tissue taken for analysis from the placenta. There is a risk of miscarriage.
- **Amniocentesis** at 14–18 weeks detects chromosomal disorders such as Down's, neural tube defects or genetic disorders and takes amniotic fluid for analysis. However, the results aren't available for around five weeks. There is a 1 per cent risk of miscarriage.

Your birth plan

Many women fear labour – whether it will go well, how they will cope with the pain. For women with epilepsy this may have special relevance if the prospect of losing control includes worry about having a seizure during labour. This does not happen often – tonic-clonic seizures occur during labour in just 1–2 per cent of women with epilepsy and within 24 hours of delivery in another 1–2 per cent. Rest assured that if this does happen, doctors and midwives will cope.

The risk of seizures during labour can be minimized by making sure you take your drugs as normal throughout labour, and that labour does not go on so long that you become exhausted, especially in the second stage – this may mean an assisted delivery, such as forceps.

You may find it helpful to include such concerns in your birth plan, which you can discuss with your midwife and other medical carers. Most women are encouraged to make a birth plan covering issues such as the type of delivery, pain relief and where to give birth – even though on the day things may not always go to plan!

- **Where to give birth.** Most women with epilepsy have straightforward deliveries, and if you feel strongly about home birth, it's best to discuss it early on in pregnancy. Home birth is not usually advised as women with epilepsy are at a slightly higher risk of complications during delivery.

- **Pain relief.** Epidural, which blocks sensation completely in the midbody, is generally felt to be safe, but be sure to tell the anaesthetist about your epilepsy and medication. TENS (transcutaneous electrical neural stimulation) is also safe. Pethidine may be potentially convulsant, so should be avoided. Gas and air are safe, but should be used carefully to avoid hyperventilation.

- **Birth companion.** Some research has shown that women experience less pain and have a speedier delivery with a trusted companion at hand. This can be anyone – your partner, a friend, or a family member. A birth companion can also remind you to take medication and inform any new staff who come on duty during your labour that you have epilepsy.

- **Breathing for birth.** You may want to ask your midwife if she can recommend an antenatal class which teaches breathing for delivery, especially if seizures are brought on by hyperventilation.

- **Birth position.** If you are very nervous about the possibility of a seizure, you may feel more comfortable giving birth on a birth stool or on the floor rather than on a bed.

- **Surroundings.** Some women are made uncomfortable by the bright lights and these may need adjusting, though photosensitivity will only be a problem for a minority.

- **Vitamin K.** Because some anticonvulsants (phenobarbitone, mysoline, carbamazepine and phenytoin) can cause vitamin K deficiency leading to haemorrhage of the newborn, it is recommended that women with epilepsy take 20 mg/day vitamin K by mouth for four weeks before the expected delivery date. It is also recommended that the baby has a vitamin K injection if you have been taking drugs phenytoin, carbamazepine, mysoline and phenobarbitone, and that the baby should also continue to have vitamin K drops by mouth for a week. There has been concern that vitamin K increases the risk of later leukaemia in the baby, though research suggests this is not so. However, if you are concerned, do discuss it with your medical carers.

- **What to do in the event of a seizure.** You will naturally want reassuring that the delivery team will know what to do if a seizure does happen. Your birth plan should include an account of a typical seizure, so that, if you do have a seizure, your delivery team will know if it is like your normal seizures. You may find it reassuring to discuss 'rescue medication' in the event of a seizure, such as oral clobazam or possibly rectal diazepam.

- **Vomiting in labour.** This can happen at 'transition' – when the first stage of labour, marked by regular contractions, moves into the second stage, when you feel the compulsion to bear down and push the baby out. Vomiting may lead to low anti-epileptic drug levels which may make a seizure more likely. So, if vomiting happens within one hour of your taking the drug, you should take it again.

Complications

Women with epilepsy have a slightly increased risk of complications, such as severe morning sickness, bleeding, toxaemia (raised blood pressure and protein in the urine) and early birth, along with an increased risk of haemorrhage during labour.

Induction (when birth is started artificially) happens more frequently with women with epilepsy – in one study it was over four times more common. There is also an increased risk of assisted delivery, with caesareans, forceps and vacuum extraction being used more than twice as often. Some recent research suggests that breech presentations are more common in women with epilepsy. The majority of babies turn head down (cephalic or vertex) but, in women with epilepsy, anti-epileptic drugs may possibly slow down the baby's natural turning process perhaps by slowing down limb movements.

Frightening as this may all sound, these complications are not usually serious. Some authorities also believe that, with recent advances in care, the complication rate is becoming closer to that of women without epilepsy, though the higher rate of sometimes severe pre-eclampsia still seems to be the case.

The warning signs of pregnancy, including those of pre-eclampsia, include:

- severe headache
- severe abdominal pain
- breaking of the waters

- mistiness, difficulty and blurring of vision
- vaginal bleeding.

If you experience any of these, consult your doctor or hospital immediately.

Life with a new baby

After all the expectancy and preparation, your baby has finally arrived, and, like any parent, you may be overwhelmed by the reality of this tiny new person in your life. Give yourself time to get over the massive impact of nine months of pregnancy followed by birth on your body.

It is important to make sure you get enough rest and sleep and to accept help from anyone who offers. Avoid too many visitors – ask your partner or other close friend to monitor them if need be. Everyone needs time alone with their new baby in the first few days, and, if your seizures are made worse by lack of sleep, you may need to explore ways of dealing with broken nights. If your seizures are controlled, one possibility may be to let your baby sleep with you in your bed – with practice, it is much easier to feed your baby while half-asleep and then drift off to sleep again without all the bother of getting up and waking up properly. Research has shown that sleeping with your baby only poses a danger to the baby if parents are heavily drugged or have taken a lot of alcohol; if you are concerned about how your anti-epileptic drugs affect you, or whether this would be safe for you, consult your doctor.

Otherwise you could ask your partner to give expressed or formula feeds by bottle at night; or arrange for a friend or family member to come in during the day so you can catch up on your sleep.

Apart from triggering seizures, being overtired can sometimes slip into postnatal depression (PND), although studies show that women with epilepsy do not seem more at risk from PND than others. Symptoms of PND include feeling you can't cope, irritability – sometimes extreme – tearfulness, sleep disturbances and appetite changes. See your doctor – PND is easily treated with modern antidepressants such as SSRIs, and the earlier you get help, the better. Support is also available from groups (see Useful addresses).

Seizures after birth can sometimes change in nature or frequency, sometimes happening more often as your body readjusts after pregnancy and delivery, so you may need to discuss having your medication readjusted.

One point about the first few weeks – as they are exposed to your drugs in the womb, very rarely babies show signs of drug withdrawal after birth, such as irritability, overactivity, restlessness, insomnia and diarrhoea, usually if you are on phenobarbitone. This may take a few weeks to settle.

Meanwhile, breastfeeding, apart from anything else, is a good way to wean your baby off the drug as he or she will receive minute amounts of the drug in your milk. The advantages of breastfeeding are that it is generally best for baby and very convenient. It can take a few weeks to establish – research shows that most women who abandon breastfeeding do so within the first month.

Sore nipples are a common early reason for giving up and can be treated with a camomile-based cream such as Kamillosan – some have found Savoy cabbage leaves helpful, as they give off an enzyme supposed to be soothing to nipples.

Sometimes high doses of certain drugs – phenobarbitone, primidone or the benzodiazepines – can make babies drowsy and slow to suck in the first days. If this happens you should see your doctor, though alternating bottle and breast feeds usually solves the problem.

Babycare and safety

When I had Bethan my husband was at sea – away three months, home three months. I was having several seizures a day but never dropped the baby. Although I have no recollection of putting her on the settee it almost seemed to be instinctive. I would come round lying on the floor but the baby was always on the settee or in the pram. I was alone but I wasn't frightened.
Janice

Again, you can discuss safety issues with your midwife, health visitor or doctor. Controlled epilepsy should not interfere with your ability to look after a baby. Newborns are tougher than they look and a few simple precautions will help minimize the risk of any accidents to your baby if you tend to have sudden seizures without warning.

- Feed and change the baby on the floor. It may be reassuring to sit propped against lots of cushions and beanbags, or against a wall or chair to avoid falling on the baby if you have a seizure.
- Bathtime is an especially delightful part of the day with your baby so

don't let others persuade you to miss out on safety grounds; just make sure someone else is around. Babies don't need bathing every day, so topping and tailing with cotton wool, flannel or sponge will be fine on other occasions.

- Keep hot drinks at a safe distance from your baby.
- If you're nervous about carrying your baby, keep him in a pram and have cuddles on the floor instead.

Further safety advice is available from epilepsy support organizations.

Enjoying your baby

As with epilepsy at other times, overprotection can be a risk – of you during pregnancy, and of the baby once he or she is born. It can sometimes happen that new mothers, with the best of intentions from others, are persuaded out of much personal care of your baby for fear of having a seizure. It is well known that the new mother does need mothering. Help is always welcome with a baby, and too many mothers struggle on in isolation, with very little relief from often remote families.

But, babies are not small for long, and the first year is a prime time for forming close emotional bonds that will last for life, and for gaining confidence in motherhood as you learn more and more about your baby and how to care for her. Not only are babies delightful and charming company. Many women, with or without epilepsy, surprise themselves at how capable and resourceful they become through the process of looking after them. Too much interference from others can stop this natural personal growth that takes place as women become mothers.

To gain confidence, you may find it useful to talk to other mothers, with or without epilepsy, about life with a new baby (see Useful addresses). It can sometimes be easy to blame epilepsy for all difficulties, when in fact settling down with a new arrival is a huge emotional upheaval which may need several months and lots of support before you really adjust. It does take time for any mother to learn how to look after a new baby, but, like any life challenge, it is something which can only really be lived through by you.

7

Everyday healthy living – looking after yourself

Looking after yourself in daily life can often be key in seizure control. While lifestyle changes may not cure epilepsy, they may sometimes be the factor which helps reduce seizure frequency or severity. Because epilepsy is so individual, what people find useful varies. This chapter looks at several different lifestyle measures which different people have found effective, including stress management, diet and nutrition, social drinking, breathing and meditation, and hobbies which can have therapeutic value, such as music and gardening.

A study of 23 people who had rejected drug therapy looked at other non-drug treatments, one of the main ones being 'life hygiene' or avoidance of seizure triggers such as lack of sleep or too much alcohol. Eight of the 23 were completely seizure-free after four years. The study concluded that treatments can be useful for people with milder forms of epilepsy, though most doctors would probably add, in conjunction with your usual drug regime. If you feel that improving your lifestyle improves your epilepsy and you want to reduce medication, do discuss it with your doctor first.

Apart from seizure control, there has been growing emphasis on quality of life for people with epilepsy. The original anticonvulsants, such as bromide, controlled seizures but effectively made people into zombies. Since then, the emphasis in epilepsy treatment has traditionally been on seizure control. More recent anti-epileptic drugs appear to have much less in the way of side effects. There has also been growing recognition of the fact that enjoying life to the full is as important as controlling seizures, and sometimes more so. By raising your energy level and improving your general health, changes in lifestyle may boost your zest in life – in itself well worth aiming for.

Dealing with stress

Centuries ago, stress described the amount of physical torture required to extract a confession, according to stress expert Dr David Lewis. Medieval inquisitors used thumbscrews to exert compression stress, the rack produced tensile stress, while the Iron Maiden's spikes applied sheer stress! The view of stress as torture certainly still lingers on today, especially among those with epilepsy who have been taught from an early age to regard stress as something to be dreaded in case it causes a seizure. However, stress can be a friend, used correctly. It's a bit like salt – while too much is deadly, the right amount adds flavour to life, helping you attain peak alertness so that you function better. Don't forget that boredom too can bring on seizures! Also, it may not actually be the stress which causes seizures, but the way you react – for example, stress may make you lose sleep or neglect your diet, so putting your body under pressure. Learning to deal with epilepsy and any associated stresses can make you healthier as you learn what your body can and cannot accept.

Causes of stress may be:

- **physical** – being tensed up, not eating properly, not getting enough sleep, drinking too much, not taking enough exercise;
- **psychological** – emotional upsets, confrontations, deadlines, lack of money, housing problems, job worries – you name it!

You will probably find your self-esteem is higher if you can manage rather than avoid stress, and there are many ways to do it. The rest of this chapter suggests ways to improve lifestyle which can only have a beneficial effect on stress, but, also, you may want to use the following suggestions to help make you more aware of exactly what causes you stress.

- **Identify key stressors.** This might be certain relationships, or work situations, and they may be big or small.

  Janice would start feeling tense when her husband was due to arrive home from work because his return meant that the relative freedom she enjoyed during the day would now be curtailed. Daphne always felt her heart starting to thud when she had to attend three-hour meetings at work in the conference room, which had no windows. Anthea, a nurse, would become progressively more stressed during the day as the clinic got busier and busier and other people seemed to heap more and more on her. Alan got on well with everyone at work except the person he worked with most – this personality clash made him feel almost physically uncomfortable.

- **Keep a stress diary for a week** to see if your stress levels are affected by any circumstances. This could be diet, lack of sleep, or just your daily biological rhythm – some people are more vulnerable at certain times of the day due to changes in this rhythm. For example, many people experience a dip in energy in the mid-afternoon, or later in the evening. Also, write down any stress feelings you experience such as thudding heart, dry mouth, tense shoulders, headache and so on.

- **Make a stress-busting plan.** Now that you've identified what causes you stress, decide what action to take and stick to it for a month. You may need to talk to someone about any anxieties. You could try improving your diet and taking more exercise. Making changes at work is another possibility, such as making sure you get away from the work environment during your lunch hour. Some people have also found it very therapeutic to take up new activities, such as music or gardening (see below, Music therapy and Horticultural therapy).

Diet

Since the ancient Greeks, epilepsy has always been treated with special diets, usually combined with other lifestyle measures such as regular hours and enough exercise. A healthy diet lowers stress, and builds up resistance to illness, another time when people are more vulnerable to seizures. Eating properly is also important because occasionally lack of food can set off a seizure. Finally, some people feel that their epilepsy is linked to nutrient shortages and/or allergic reactions to some foods and other substances, although when investigated medically such claims often cannot be substantiated.

Many of these factors will be tackled by eating a diet which follows basic well-known healthy eating rules – planning meals around complex carbohydrates such as rice and pasta, avoiding processed and refined foods, cutting right down on fat and sugar, and having plenty of fresh fruit and vegetables. Make sure you eat a variety of foods from the four key food groups – milk and dairy products; bread and cereals; fruit and vegetables; and protein such as meat, fish and poultry – in other words, a healthy diet.

Keeping blood sugar levels steady

Seizures have been linked with low blood sugar or hypoglycaemia (hypo means low, glycaemia means blood sugar). Mood swings, which affect some people with epilepsy, and pre-menstrual tension, have also occasionally been linked with low blood sugar, as have other conditions which can have an adverse effect on people with epilepsy, such as stress, panic attacks, migraine and insomnia. It seems that sudden drops do most harm, and also that people can suffer symptoms if levels are unstable rather than abnormally low – that is, the levels are within normal limits but still fluctuate enough to affect you.

Symptoms of low blood sugar include anxiety and stress symptoms such as palpitations, headaches, feeling shaky, waking in the small hours and finding it hard to drop off again, energy dips mid-morning and mid-afternoon, wanting to eat again around an hour after the evening meal, not wanting breakfast, and physical symptoms including twitching eyelids.

What causes low blood sugar? When food is eaten, glucose from the food passes into the bloodstream, where your body uses it for energy. If the glucose level rises too high, the pancreas tends to flood the body with insulin to bring it down. You then crave more sugar – and so the cycle goes on. Over a long period, the pancreas risks becoming exhausted, so that the whole process works less effectively, while you need more and more sugar, and may feel less and less well. Other factors apart from food can stress the pancreas so that it overproduces insulin – exercise, stress, pregnancy and the effect of some drugs.

We do need sugar – in fact the brain is dependent on it – but it needs to be the right sort, not refined, instantly absorbed carbohydrates in the form of sweets, cakes or white bread. The brain is dependent on glucose and would die without it, as, unlike muscle tissue, it cannot use other foods such as protein. This is why there are so many symptoms of altered brain chemistry when the blood sugar level drops quickly. A brain short of glucose is a brain short of oxygen – on an everyday level, you may have noticed how you yawn when you go for too long without food, and bounce back with renewed energy after you have eaten.

Managing blood sugar

- Eat at regular intervals and don't go for more than three hours without food. Keep portions small if you're concerned about weight.
- Try and have breakfast, such as fruit, unsweetened fruit juice, porridge, unsugared muesli, wholemeal toast, crispbread, rice cakes, grilled bacon, eggs, mushrooms, tomatoes.
- Make sure you have snacks mid-morning and mid-afternoon, such as a handful of sunflower seeds and raisins, yoghurt or an apple – the pectin is said to be a good blood sugar level stabilizer.
- Also have a snack last thing before going to bed – a milk drink can help boost calcium levels as well as helping you get to sleep.

- Avoid or cut down on refined carbohydrates such as sugar, chocolate, sweets, cakes, biscuits, sugary drinks, white flour, white bread, processed and packet food, and junk food.
- Eat unrefined complex carbohydrates such as whole grain cereals, wheat, oats, barley rice, rye millet, wholemeal bread, wholemeal pasta, potatoes, brown rice, beans, lentils, chickpeas, nuts, seeds.
- Include lots of fresh vegetables and fruit, with meals and as snacks. These are absorbed more slowly by the body and will provide essential vitamins and minerals which can be depleted by regular drug-taking.

Points about protein

Many nutritionists say we eat too much protein – others, not enough! The effect of protein may vary from person to person. Some people find that including more protein in their diet helps control low blood sugar, boost energy, and even lose weight. Protein may also help you get rid of excess water, important especially for women who tend to suffer bloating and water retention before a period, which can affect seizure control. Good sources of protein include meat, fish, eggs, cheese, pulses such as peas and beans, and nuts.

A possible link between seizures and amino acids, chemicals which make up proteins, has been established by researchers at the University of California. The scientists found that diets deficient in amino acids can make seizures more likely in rats. While the study highlights the importance of ensuring that people everywhere eat an adequate level of high-quality protein, it does not suggest supplementing your diet with amino acids as a treatment for epilepsy in most cases. However, some individuals have tried this with reported success. Taurine, an amino acid which helps inhibit neuronal activity, has been tried in sometimes mega-doses by some people with epilepsy, who have found it does help control their seizures, though if you are going to experiment it is probably wiser to start with small doses and build up, and also to check with your doctor first. DMG (Di-methyl glycine) is another amino acid which helps oxygen move round the system and is said to stimulate the immune system.

Paul suffered from repeated absence seizures, and the occasional tonic-clonic seizure. Paul saw a nutritionist and was recommended supplements of about 90 mg of DMG twice a day, which he bought in a health food shop. He took it for about a year, and then found he didn't seem to need it any more as he no longer suffered from seizures. In his case, DMG did seem to be a miracle cure, but it is well recognized that many people can 'grow out' of their absence seizures.

The right nutrients

As Paul's story suggests, certain nutritional deficiencies may be particularly associated with epilepsy, and, in people with a low seizure threshold, may make epilepsy worse. While true deficiencies are rare, it may well be that improving your diet generally will make you feel better.

Some anti-epileptic drugs deplete nutrients, particularly folic acid and vitamin D. Supplements should be discussed with your doctor, as, depending on your drugs, you may need to check that what you are intending to take won't unbalance your nutrient levels further.

Nutrient shortages which have been suggested as rarely implicated with seizures include the following.

- *Calcium* shortage (hypocalcaemia) though rare, has been identified as a metabolic disorder especially in newborns. Low calcium has also been associated with seizures in some medical studies, including ones which looked at coeliac disease (see below), which may cause calcium to be lost from the body, though this too is not common. The body does need calcium for the smooth running of the central nervous system, and lack of it has also been associated with pre-menstrual symptoms such as irritability, muscle cramps and fluid retention. The best sources of calcium are milk and dairy products, bony fish (i.e. sardines), seeds, nuts (especially almonds), dried figs, bread and dark green leafy vegetables.

- *Vitamin B6* (pyridoxine) deficiency is a recognized but rare source of seizures in newborns. Some research suggests it very rarely produces convulsions in adults, and possibly causes pre-seizure symptoms such as irritability, sensitivity to noise, and abnormal EEGs. It is probably best not to take B6 alone as it increases the need for other B vitamins, particularly B2 and pantothenic acid, so it may be best taken as vitamin B complex. Good sources of vitamin B6 include meat, whole grains and pulses.

- *Folic acid* deficiency is made worse by some anti-epileptic drugs, but it may be dangerous to supplement this on your own as it has been suggested that large doses of folic acid can make epilepsy worse. Eat folate-rich foods such as fruit, dark leafy vegetables, other veg such as broccoli, cereals, pulses and yeast extract.

- *Vitamin D*, which helps the body absorb calcium, is found in most oil fish and some animal products, especially in cheese and fortified milks; and vitamin E, important for boosting oxygen flow round the body.

- *Zinc* is important for brain functioning and helps raise levels of taurine in the brain. It works best in combination with manganese. Zinc is found in meat and offal, wheatgerm, nuts, crab, oysters and lentils.

- *Magnesium* shortage has also rarely been linked with seizures. Magnesium is found in wholemeal flour, millet, figs, meat, fish, nuts and pulses.

- *Manganese* – some research suggests that eating more manganese during pregnancy may help prevent seizures in the baby, though this is not completely proved. Good sources of manganese include rice, wholemeal bread, wheatgerm, buckwheat, lima beans, nuts, cockles, sardines, blackberries, figs and pineapple.

Reacting to foods and the environment

Some people with a low seizure threshold have found that paying attention to particular foods and environmental factors can make a difference to their seizures – sometimes a dramatic one.

Julie found that cutting out caffeine completely resulted in a very considerable reduction in her seizures – from 77 to 17 in one year. Daphne found she felt much better for eating organic food where possible, peeling all fruit and vegetables, and drinking filtered or mineral water. Anthea, who also suffered from migraines, found her wellbeing and seizure control improved when she cut out red wine, cheese, strawberries and seafood.

Allergy is a debated issue – some doctors say it is much less common than most people believe; others say it is a sign of a poor diet which is deficient in nutrients; yet others believe allergy is a natural reaction to an increasingly toxic environment.

How do you tell if you are allergic to food? Apart from obvious reactions like a seizure or feeling dreadful, allergy may be more likely if you tend to suffer from other allergy-related conditions such as asthma, eczema and hayfever.

Common food allergens include:

- wheat and other gluten-containing foods such as rye, barley, oats, buckwheat, and prepared foods containing these ingredients. Wheat allergy is usually viewed as causing coeliac disease, often linked with epilepsy, when the body is prevented from absorbing nutrients (malabsorption syndrome) by persistent diarrhoea, vomiting and poor appetite. It is thought to be due to an inability to digest wheat gluten, which contains an intestinal irritant, gliadin. Coeliac disease may put people at greater risk of seizures because nutrients such as iron and calcium are more easily lost.
- milk and dairy products
- sugar and artificial sweeteners such as aspartame
- eggs
- peanuts
- fruits such as citrus fruit and strawberries
- shellfish
- food additives and preservatives

Social drinking

Some people with epilepsy prefer not to drink at all, but many do enjoy going out with friends to the pub or having a glass of wine at dinner. This shouldn't be a problem though you may want to double-check with your doctor if you can safely drink on your current anti-epileptic medication and if so, how much.

Research suggests that drinking more than two units of alcohol in less than 12–15 hours significantly increases the risk of seizures in people with epilepsy. (A unit of alcohol is a half-pint of beer or cider, a glass of wine or sherry, or one measure of spirits such as whisky or gin.)

Sometimes it is not so much the alcohol as how it is drunk – that is, if it forms part of late nights, missed meals, or forgotten tablets, all of which can make seizures more likely. Some people don't take their drugs while drinking as a precaution against a seizure but it is more important to take your medication as usual and drink moderately. It can also be important to look after yourself after drinking, as many seizures take place after alcohol has been consumed due to alcohol withdrawal. So, it may be helpful to arrange for a lie-in after a particularly demanding social evening!

While it is much more socially acceptable not to drink these days, especially with drink-drive campaigns, it is possible to join in the fun without making it obvious you're drinking less than others. Ploys include drinking alcohol-free wine or beer, taking half-pints instead of pints, or mixing beer or wine with soft drinks such as lemonade.

Moderate wine drinking may be better than beer or cider if you are taking carbamazepine, because people on this drug are less able to deal with large amounts of fluid, which may occasionally be dangerous as it can cause water intoxication.

Photosensitive epilepsy

Watching television and video or using computers can affect a minority of people with epilepsy. This can be detected on an EEG. It is usually adolescent girls who have seizures precipitated by flashing lights. This problem can be life long but drugs such as sodium valproate are good at stopping the sensitivity to flashing lights. The following recommendations may be helpful.

- Make sure your posture is comfortable, and restrict your viewing if need be.
- View the TV in a well-lit room.
- Sit at least 2.5 metres away and at an angle from the television.
- Use a high-frequency TV (100Mhz).
- Make sure your TV is working properly as faulty screens can cause problems.
- Some photosensitive reactions can be minimized by covering one eye.
- Special TV sunglasses are also available via epilepsy support organizations.
- Use an American video screen for computers.

Breathing and meditation

Correct breathing may be useful to help control stress feelings and fear of having a seizure, especially if seizures are brought on by hyperventilation. You may also want to think about breathing if you are a woman preparing for birth – childbirth expert Sheila Kitzinger has some useful advice on this (see Further reading).

First, try and be aware of how you breathe. Because of stress and tension we often slip into incorrect breathing habits without realizing it. This is often due to poor posture including bad habits of sitting, standing and walking, so that our shoulders become tensed up, the head pulled back, and the chest narrowed, which means we can't breathe to our full capacity. This can affect the circulation so that not enough oxygen gets to the brain.

Two remedies which are very useful for posture and breathing are yoga and the Alexander Technique. An Indian study, published in the *Indian Journal of Medical Research*, found that yoga and meditation significantly reduced seizures in patients by as much as 86 per cent. Alexander aims to help people relearn correct posture. Again, see Further reading for suggestions on where to find out more about both therapies, though you will probably gain more benefit if you can attend a class in person.

- **Coping with hyperventilation**. Place a paper bag (not a plastic one) over your mouth and nose and breathe into it. Hyperventilation means getting too much oxygen in from the air so as you breathe in the carbon dioxide you have just expelled this will help balance your breathing. Or, splash your face and hands with cold water.

- **Energizing breath**. Alternate nostril breathing is said to charge the two halves of the brain, so leading to overall neurological and physical balance and raising the energy. Close your right nostril with your right thumb and inhale through your left nostril. Hold for a few seconds, then exhale through your right nostril, closing the left nostril with the ring finger of your right hand. Now inhale through the right nostril; hold, and exhale through the left nostril. Repeat for a minute or two.

- **Calming breath**. Lie comfortably on your back and inhale to a count of ten, making sure you take the breath in via your abdomen and then up into your chest. Pause for a second or two, then exhale slowly to a count of ten. You can do this sitting up, or standing, whenever you feel tense or stressed.

- **The Om factor!** In Transcendental Meditation (TM), a personal mantra is used for meditation which is supposed to be personally revealed by a teacher of TM to each student. However, it is usually Om. In Hinduism, Om represents the most sacred and comprehensive expression of spiritual knowledge. An easy and effective form of meditation simply involves listening to yourself say Om silently or aloud. After several minutes, you may find that you reach a deep and soothing level of consciousness in which daily petty irritations can be left behind.

Music therapy

'I fall sick when I hear the sound of the street vendor's flute in the evening sun, although I do not know the reason,' said the Chinese poet Kung Tsu Chen, writing in 1847. He is describing a rare form of reflex epilepsy, musicogenic epilepsy, which affects an estimated 1 in 10 million. Seizures may occur on hearing the music, or even while thinking or dreaming of music, and may take several seconds or even minutes to develop. They appear to be most common in the right temporal lobe, which houses the right auditory cortex, an area implicated in the processing of melody.

There may be another side to the coin. Some recent research suggests that music can reduce seizures as well as inducing them. One study, reported in *Clinical Electroencephalography*, found that some music seemed to reduce seizures. The researchers studied 29 people with frequent seizures, either awake or in coma, and found that 23 of them had a significant drop in seizures, with an average reduction in seizure rate from 62 per cent to 21 per cent. The effect was confined to Mozart's music – pop music made no difference. Moreover, the music was effective in patients who were in a comatose state, so presumably not consciously aware of the music.

The so-called 'Mozart effect' has figured in a number of other studies looking at how music affects the brain, especially as boosting mathematical and other intellectual abilities. While it is too early to speculate about using music as a treatment for epilepsy, it may well be that including more music in your daily life could be beneficial. It could also boost confidence to learn an instrument or join a choir, not least for the fact of being with other people. Singing can help loosen the ribs, chest muscles, and the anterior, middle and posterior scalene muscles where the neck joins the shoulders, so helping release tension and stress, and making breathing deeper and more regular. A Swedish study of nearly 13,000 people found that those who join in musical activities such as choirs tend to live longer – definitely worth a try!

Art therapy

Because it doesn't use words, art can be an especially soothing and therapeutic way of releasing feelings, something which many people with or without epilepsy find difficult. It may be especially helpful in dealing with stress, or if you feel you're 'stuck' generally in life, as it often allows unconscious messages to emerge.

Art therapy is now increasingly used for relationship difficulties, or to boost self-esteem – both of which can be key for people with epilepsy just as for other people. It may also help those who have learning difficulties in addition to epilepsy, who often have even more than the normal trouble expressing their emotions effectively, and some of whom, in their frustration, may resort to less mature ways of showing their feelings such as banging or shouting.

Some therapists offer a mix of art therapy and counselling to help people analyse their drawings and paintings. Therapists may, for example, look at why you have drawn yourself as a tiny figure in the corner and your partner as a huge giant covering the rest of the page! Colour has special significance too, which is usually fairly obvious even though people may not really be aware of it at the time of painting: red may represent passion or anger, blue coldness, black, sadness or endings.

Needless to say you don't need any artistic skill though you may be surprised, under tuition, at the artistic competency which does emerge. Contrary perhaps to common assumptions, art can be taught.

Horticultural therapy

Horticultural therapy is based on the so-called biophilia effect – the love of living things. Like art therapy, it doesn't depend on using words, which again can be useful for those who find it hard to express or intellectualize their feelings. However, it may differ from other art forms which are made but not nurtured in the same way – dealing with a growing, live object over a long period.

For people with epilepsy, horticultural therapy may have special significance in terms of taking responsibility. It may also help some people think more effectively about time management, as raising plants demands planning over a period of time, sowing at certain times, and waiting for results.

Just being outside may be as helpful as anything. Research by biologists has found that natural daylight is vital for the normal functioning of the brain, the smooth running of the central nervous system, and the sleep–wake cycle.

8

Practical issues

There are certain subjects which are likely to get a rather enflamed response from many people with epilepsy, who feel that they face more than their fair share of the usual hurdles in achieving what they want. Take work, for example. Ask most employers what their attitude to epilepsy is, and you are likely to get a positive, polite response. Most people are eager to appear liberal and tolerant! And, many employers are indeed sympathetic to people with epilepsy. Nevertheless, some are less so, and, in today's difficult job market, it helps to be as prepared as possible when it comes to tackling the thorny question of gaining and keeping paid work.

> I graduated from an Open University BA course in philosophy, with a year off while my medication was changed from Tegretol to topiramate. When I took my finals I had two seizures the morning of the exam and one the night before, and so did the papers with a black eye and cut chin! The OU were fantastic – faxing my GP and being very understanding. With the degree in my pocket, I felt ready for anything the world of work could throw at me.
> *Gloria*

Most people with epilepsy should have no trouble attaining whatever educational standards they set themselves. It may take more preparation and paperwork, but, as Jan's story shows, it is possible to take a degree on your own terms. Perhaps one of the strongest problems is inner lack of confidence rather than attitudes from others, and you may find it helpful to look for help here, such as counselling to boost self-esteem, or more specific advice from a careers advisor.

Legislation plays a part in work – some jobs are barred from people with epilepsy on safety grounds – and in driving, the other issue which has great significance for people with epilepsy. Driving laws, also made on safety grounds, are a source of much frustration among people with epilepsy. However, driving laws have been somewhat relaxed over the past few years, with the required seizure-free interval going down from two years to one.

With activities too, another area which can cause disagreement especially among people uninformed about epilepsy, there is growing recognition that many people with epilepsy may enjoy as much freedom as other people. Safety, often used as an excuse to wrap the person with epilepsy in cotton wool by overprotective others, can also be approached in a more relaxed way, a few common-sense precautions usually being sufficient for the majority of people with epilepsy.

Your career

Research is conflicting when it comes to work and epilepsy, perhaps because of the divide (mentioned above) between what employers put down on paper, and what happens in practice. For example, a recent survey for the UK's Institute of Employment Studies found that epilepsy is one of a group of conditions that employers see as least likely to cause problems, and is viewed on a par with hearing problems, allergies and skin conditions, heart and circulation problems and diabetes.

Other research suggests that careers advisors often consider epilepsy to be the most difficult condition, after mental illness, to place in employment. Following the Disability Discrimination Act of 1996, one survey found that epilepsy came top at 78 per cent of conditions considered to be a disability under the Act, closely followed by colour blindness and schizophrenia!

While many employers are sympathetic, a number of others still have outdated ideas about the condition. Common misapprehensions are that epilepsy is a sign of lower intelligence or a violent personality; or that you must call a doctor for all seizures. As Bronwen put it, 'Ignorance is the problem you have to deal with; not prejudice.'

One of the main stumbling blocks is the idea that all epilepsy is the same. 'A common mistake when considering people with epilepsy for employment is to make sweeping generalisations about what they can and cannot do,' states the GP Information and Educational Resource. While it may seem blindingly obvious that there is a huge difference between someone whose epilepsy has been under control for ten years, and someone who is having several seizures a day, employers with little or no experience of epilepsy may sometimes not discriminate. Or again, there may be little recognition of the fact that ongoing seizures are not necessarily always a bar to employment, or that willing employers can and do often get round this with a little adjustment, such as making allowances for the occasional epilepsy-related absence from work, or learning to cope with the odd seizure at work without panicking and calling an ambulance.

As with medical treatment, people with epilepsy need to be considered on an individual basis when employment is in question. Some jobs are precluded by law, and however outdated and unfair you consider this, there is little that can be done short of campaigning for a change in legislation, perhaps with an epilepsy support group. Bear in mind too that traditional job structures have changed or are fast changing, so that some people may want to consider other options, such as working from home or self-employment.

Ideally, people with epilepsy should be considered in the light of their experience and qualifications first, and in terms of their epilepsy second. The main question you will probably need to consider is how predictable seizures are and what they consist of – how controlled they are; whether you have an aura; whether there is any pattern to seizures or if they occur at a particular time of day, such as on first awakening; and whether you have any common triggers, such as too little sleep or too much alcohol, or, less commonly, specific triggers such as the sound of machinery.

Audrey suffered from musicogenic epilepsy (described in Chapter 7), a very rare form of reflex epilepsy, in which a person reacts to a very specific stimulus with a seizure. Her epilepsy was triggered by certain notes of music, and the sound of bells or ringing sounds, which made getting a job very difficult indeed because of the telephone. She finally abandoned office work, which she had continued with after the car accident which had caused her epilepsy, and became a house-matron in a school for children with epilepsy.

Applying for a job and disclosing epilepsy

Anyone may benefit from having an expert eye cast over his or her CV, and many specialist companies exist which can help update a CV and present your qualifications in the best possible light.

Filling in an application form can be awkward if you have to fill in a medical questionnaire which effectively forces you to reveal epilepsy at that point, say by ticking a box. The ideal would be for disclosure to take place at a time of your choosing, not someone else's. However, legally, there is no option, though instead of just ticking the box it is important to enclose a covering letter with the form. The covering letter should be relatively short – no more than one A4 side – and typed if at all possible. It should explain:

- how epilepsy affects you individually, and in particular how predictable it is in terms of being seizure-free or having seizures with an aura, a particular pattern, or with specific triggers;
- why the epilepsy should not be a problem for this particular job;
- whether you have or are eligible for a driving licence. 'The driving licence is a great advantage. It shows that the government is willing to license the person to drive a vehicle that kills and injures thousands of people each year on our roads. This should suggest to a potential employer that the person is safe in most work environments', according to the GP Information and Educational Resource.

Disclosing epilepsy at interview has more potential advantages as the employer has a chance to see you and talk to you, rather than judging you from a letter. You also have the chance to explain verbally how epilepsy affects you in a positive, factual way. Disclosure once you've been offered the job is not usually recommended, as you can be dismissed.

Some people do not disclose their epilepsy at all when applying for a job, especially if it is well controlled or seizures only happen occasionally or at night. Disclosing epilepsy is often recommended for the sake of solidarity with others with the condition, so that they show employers how well and efficiently people with epilepsy work. This way, employed people with epilepsy may act as ambassadors for others' long-term future and improve long-term work prospects for future generations. Not everyone agrees, however. One survey showed that more than 50 per cent of those who had two or more full-time jobs had never disclosed their epilepsy to an employer, and only one in ten people had always revealed it. The same survey suggests that concealment certainly raises the chances of being employed, as employment of men with epilepsy was just 7 per cent below male workers generally (74 per cent compared with 81 per cent).

Technically, however, not disclosing epilepsy is illegal, as you risk dismissal at a later date for not disclosing the information at application stage. The whole situation, based on outdated legislation, gives people with epilepsy very little protection from the law at any stage. In the USA, for example, employers cannot ask questions about health at application stage and if they ask about them after offering a job only a person with appropriate qualifications, such as an occupational health specialist, is allowed to make the decision as to whether someone is medically fit for the job. This situation is far fairer than in the UK, where few employers have specialist health knowledge at all let alone about epilepsy, and can all too easily make decisions based on inadequate knowledge.

This really leaves people with epilepsy in a cleft stick, as at the moment there is no legal protection for people refused a job on account of their health, even if you could discover – and prove – this was the real reason, and almost no protection also for employees dismissed for their health record. This kind of discrimination often operates silently for a number of groups, such as women and older people, and is often silently put up with. How can people with epilepsy fight this?

One way is to be open about epilepsy from the start in a positive way. In general, the more information and understanding employers have the more understanding they will be; it is hard for an employer to maintain any general, vague prejudice or ignorance face to face with an individual prospective employee who is capable of giving the facts in a calm, articulate way.

The Disability Discrimination Act should in theory make a difference though discrimination is still allowed if employers can show 'good reason' for it and companies with fewer than 20 employees are exempt from the provisions of the Act. However, one person with epilepsy has won a court case for unfair dismissal under the Act, so this could be used as a precedent.

You may well not want to have to campaign for epilepsy as well as trying to get yourself a job, but, unfortunately, it is often still necessary to educate potential employers about epilepsy.

Epilepsy didn't affect my life until I decided to teach and was advised not to because of my epilepsy. Being stubborn, this made me even more determined! I didn't want to qualify to teach normal children but I eventually taught deaf children, gaining my Cert. Ed. at college as well as my TOD (Teacher of the Deaf) certificate involving speech therapy and taking audiograms. Because I have epilepsy that is not controlled I had to have two interviews with a special employment officer for the county council, who decided I should only teach when there was a nurse in the room, i.e. special education. This suited me fine as I only wanted to teach in special education but not every teacher with epilepsy will think so!
Jan

Once you've got the job

Once the major hurdle of getting the job is over, and you are safely ensconced in a work routine, there are other challenges to consider, such as making sure you are given your share of the stimulating tasks, not just the dogsbody work, and being promoted to the limits of your ability.

> I took a BSc in maths but feel I have failed myself as my career never took off. After losing two jobs in succession – I thought because of epilepsy though it can't be proved – I did jobs which could have been done by anyone with a few O levels.
> *Vicky*

Some recent surveys of working people with epilepsy have suggested that unemployment is not the major problem it was once thought to be, but that discrimination at work is a more serious problem which could lead to under-employment and restricted career development. Continuing seizures may also make it difficult to hold down a job. The other main problem is lack of special skills – as Vicky's story shows, not perhaps always skills in the sense of academic or other qualifications, but perhaps skills in getting noticed and in getting the work you want.

Here specialist advice from employment services may make a difference, including short- and long-term career planning along with practical advice on self-presentation and communication skills, as well as emotional support.

Dealing with employers' objections

While many employers are only too anxious to be politically correct and fair in their approach, some will have objections, either voiced openly as below, or more covert. The latter are harder to deal with but this is why adopting an open positive approach from the start can be helpful.

'I don't know anything about epilepsy so I don't feel justified in taking you on.'
This is blatantly lazy, and can be dealt with by a quick skim even through just one of the leaflets provided by epilepsy self-help organizations.

'I can't employ you because I don't have a nurse or other trained medical personnel.'

This is unfair and may not be justifiable under the DDA. You do not need medical personnel for first aid and anyway most companies should have at least one person with basic first aid skills.

'You'll take time off after seizures/for doctor's appointments.'
This needs dealing with on an individual basis. If you do need say a short rest after seizures, or have any other special needs, it is only fair to say so, but, this can be negotiated. It may also be worth pointing out that for example smokers on average take four minutes time off work per cigarette!

'You will alarm your colleagues if you have seizures in their company.'
Again, providing information to colleagues can be very helpful in dispelling this attitude – lack of information and understanding is often what lies behind fear and prejudice.

'You just won't achieve what I want because of your epilepsy and people will have to make excuses or cover for you.'
This is judging you in advance. In fact, surveys have shown that people with epilepsy tend to work harder, be more conscientious, and take less time off.

Driving

If you are unable to use your driving licence you do save on the hassle of car repairs and running expenses. You also tend to be fitter and healthier because you walk more.
Anthea

Most countries don't let people with epilepsy drive unless they have been seizure-free (from all seizure types, including auras, myoclonic jerks and absence seizures) for a set time which may vary widely, usually from three to eighteen months; the interval recently adopted by EEC countries including the UK is one year. In the UK, you can also drive if you have only had seizures in your sleep for the past three years. If you are applying for a licence, you must inform the DVLA (Driver and Vehicle Licensing Agency) about your epilepsy. If you already hold a licence but have a seizure, then the law states that you must also inform the DVLA, and stop driving. You then lose your licence until once again you have been seizure-free for a year.

As with other aspects of epilepsy including work, traditionally it has been usual to treat all people with epilepsy the same and to ban driving right across the board. More recently, though, it has become clear that the risks are not high for people who have controlled epilepsy. But, there is a grey area for people whose seizures are not perfectly controlled – is it safe to drive? If so, when? How do you decide?

Driving is a very important issue for people with epilepsy. It is often seen as a key area representing personal freedom, adulthood and independence. It is also an area with very practical implications in terms of being employable and just in sheer mobility, for example, if you depend on driving for a job, or live in a rural area where, as is common in the UK, public transport is woefully inadequate.

> I'll never forget those nightmare trips into town for shopping – baby plus buggy plus shopping plus rain plus waiting for the bus – plus epilepsy!
> *Daphne*

Research at Johns Hopkins University, Baltimore, and the University of Maryland, USA, has come up with certain specific risk factors which may help assess the chances of having a car accident due to seizures. The researchers hope that this approach may be more effective in reducing accident deaths than current driving policies which, the study also found, a significant number of people with epilepsy simply ignore, either by not reporting their seizures as required by law, or just by driving in spite of having continuing seizures. Only 36 per cent of the group with previous crashes and 40 per cent of the control group reported their seizures to authorities. And, more than half of the patients in the crash group and a third of the non-crash group drove despite having seizure-free intervals shorter than their states legally required.

Driving against medical advice is often a defiant reaction which seeks to deny the epilepsy. The problem is, as with some jobs, it involves others. An Australian study showed that charges of murder and manslaughter were felt to be appropriate for people who drove despite having continued seizures.

The Johns Hopkins scientists found four characteristics which could help predict accidents:

- The length of time people go without a seizure before they return to driving – the single feature most linked with crashes. Generally, the shorter the interval, the greater the likelihood of an accident. People who did not drive for a year or longer had a 93 per cent reduced risk.

- People who experience an aura also had reduced odds of crashing.
- So did people with fewer non-epilepsy-related accidents in general before they were diagnosed.
- Reducing the number of anti-epileptic drugs, or changing them, lowered the accident risk, probably because of less sedation.

Coping with driving restrictions

Frustrating as the regulations can be, they are designed with safety in mind. Some people with epilepsy feel safe driving because they always get a warning of their attacks, or because they view their seizures as minor, where their consciousness is barely disturbed. However, this doesn't take into account the fact that epilepsy is a dynamic, not a static condition. Seizures can change their nature, sometimes from one week to the next, so that the warning disappears and the minor attacks become major ones. Also, even if attacks are 'minor', it can only take a second's loss of concentration to cause an accident.

However, if you feel that your seizures hardly merit the name, for example if they are confined to a few myoclonic jerks in the morning, then you can apply for advice to the DVLA's medical unit. This is open to anyone who disagrees with refusal to grant him or her a licence because of epilepsy, and the matter may be referred to a specialist for an informed, balanced decision to be made.

Again, you may feel that your attacks are not epileptic in nature and that there is nothing to stop you driving; in which case you may need to seek a further opinion (see Chapter 3 for more on the diagnostic procedure).

If you are not currently eligible for a licence, you can ask your doctor to help you cope with your changed circumstances by writing a letter to your employer which can be used to back up a request for a change of job within the same company. The letter does not have to state that you have epilepsy, only that you are currently not able to drive for medical reasons, and not likely to be able to drive for some time. This has worked successfully for many people, though obviously it is more likely to be successful in a large, versatile company.

Another point which frequently concerns people is whether they should move house if they live in a rural area with little public transport. If your seizures seem likely to be easily controlled, then it may well be best to stay where you are and struggle through the inconvenience than uproot everyone – unless of course you want to move anyway. Ask your doctor for as much information as possible about the likelihood of seizure control so you can make an informed decision.

Exercise and activities

Quite a lot of palaver is made about activities such as rock-climbing and scuba-diving for people with epilepsy, as though everyone else were rushing off to do these every day. In practice, most people might be as concerned about finding money for these activities as safety. However, they represent freedom of activity for people with epilepsy – the fact that they should be able to do them if they want to.

Most people with epilepsy can tackle a wide range of activities with success and enjoyment, including rock-climbing! (Apparently, as one girl with epilepsy pointed out, the ropes are there to stop everyone falling off, not just people with epilepsy.) Generally, there are very few activities which the person with epilepsy cannot do. Acceptance of your limitations should be carefully considered, and, rather than accepting that you must be significantly limited by seizures, solutions can be sought to make the most of your potential.

Three factors do need to be taken into account – how safe the activity is in general, how controlled the epilepsy is, and whether any extra help or supervision is needed. Like so much else in epilepsy, this needs to be tackled on an individual basis, and discussed with activity leaders if necessary.

Swimming, a great exercise, is a common source of confusion. In fact, people are more likely to drown through not being able to swim than because of a seizure, especially in a lifeguard-supervised situation. (Drowning can also happen at home, in the bath.) Sensible precautions can help, such as swimming with a friend, staying in the shallow end, and telling the lifeguard that you have epilepsy.

Whatever form of exercise you choose, it will help you keep it up if it is something which can easily be incorporated into your current lifestyle – for example, if you pass the swimming pool on your way to the shops, or if you're lucky enough to have a gym on your work premises. To gain the maximum benefit, exercise needs to be done regularly and often, three times a week if possible.

Safety

A survey by the Epilepsy Federation of America found that women with epilepsy were more susceptible to burns. Almost one in four people (23 per cent) with epilepsy who completed a questionnaire about burns injuries reported seizure-related burns. Seventy per cent of them were women, and almost half of those with burns had complex partial seizures; 33 per cent had generalized seizures. Cooking and smoking were the most dangerous activities. Stove-top cooking accounted for 41.8 per cent of the burns, with cigarettes blamed for 20 per cent. Hot showers, ironing, campfires, room heaters and curling irons accounted for the rest. Fatigue, lack of sleep, stress and missed medication were cited as contributing factors to the seizures which led to burns.

This all illustrates the importance of looking after yourself as an important component to seizure control and general quality of life, as already stated in Chapter 7.

However, this does not mean wrapping yourself in cotton wool! Fear of injury is a major component in overprotection. It can be hard to strike the right balance. A diagnosis of epilepsy can leave people and their families scared and confused about which activities they can safely continue with and which not. An important part of this is realistically assessing risks on an individual basis.

Otherwise, it might help to adopt common safety politics which everyone would benefit from. The majority of accidents take place in the home, and much can be done to make this a safer area – something which you might need to consider anyway if you have small children or are planning to start a family. Safety suggestions include the following.

- Refit bathroom and lavatory doors so they open outwards so that the door will not be blocked if you fall behind it.
- Fit safety glass in shower cubicles and doors.
- If using a shower, make sure it is one with an efficient heat control, i.e. which cannot be turned to the warmest setting accidentally.
- Use a cooker guard with pan handles turned inwards. Serve up at the stove rather than carry boiling saucepans to the table. A microwave can be safer than a conventional oven.
- Use fire or radiator guards and avoid freestanding heaters.
- Some people move furniture to the walls of the room so the centre is more free. It is also possible to pad chairs, tables and bed bases to blend in with the room's decor.

For more advice, contact The Royal Society for the Prevention of Accidents (RoSPA; see Useful addresses).

9

Epilepsy and your feelings

To suffer from epilepsy is to be different from one's fellows as the result of a persistent, intangible and recalcitrant disorder which even in the most enlightened society carries with it a stigma of the unusual. The subject nearly always feels different from his contemporaries, and the more intelligent and enlightened he is, and the more understanding and enlightened his contemporaries, the bigger the problem he has to face, for it is greater trauma to have to be consciously treated as normal than to be naturally accepted as different.

This hurtful dilemma, ranging from sentencious and embarrassing over-understanding, to miserable restriction and loneliness, pervades his life at home, at school, at work and sometimes into marriage.
Dr D. Williams, writing in the 1950s

At school I felt different even though my friends didn't treat me as such. I couldn't drink, go to clubs or parties, or even go to places like Alton Towers because of the heights of the rides. I can't even watch TV in the dark! I felt very self-conscious and it's only recently I have been able to tell people about my epilepsy without feeling embarrassed. I was convinced that no one would want a relationship with an 'epileptic' but I've been lucky so far. My parents have been really protective so that sometimes I feel like I have no life. However, my friends are brilliant. When I get upset, they help me realize that I'm just a bit different, but not enough for it to affect them or me.
Julie

These eloquent descriptions of the psychological burden of epilepsy point out that not only is 'feeling different' a major part of epilepsy – it is something which cannot always be addressed by the outside world. Since the 1950s, when the epileptologist Dr D. Williams was writing, much hard work has been done by the epilepsy movement to establish that people with epilepsy are much the same as people anywhere. Yet, for many with epilepsy, 'feeling different' can persist even when friends are accepting, employers understanding, and lovers truly appreciative of the person who happens to have seizures.

Epilepsy, unlike many other medical disorders, is a psychosocial condition as well as a medical disorder. Its invisibility most of the time, the unpredictability of seizures, and the overwhelming loss of control involved have since time immemorial been seen as a threat to social and personal order. 'To be naturally accepted as different' is an ideal which has to fight against a long cultural history of epilepsy, and how the nature of epilepsy is perceived by others.

While epilepsy is a chronic health disorder, it is unlike many other chronic conditions in that most people with epilepsy are 'normal' most of the time – except when they have a seizure, suddenly revealing themselves as 'different', something which can happen even with those whose epilepsy has been controlled for a long time. 'Epilepsy is not a continuously rough sea, but a recurrent tidal wave,' said Dr William Lennox, one of the American fathers of the modern epilepsy movement – the 'recurrent tidal wave' being the sudden unpredictable quality of the symptom of epilepsy, compared with the constant 'rough sea' of many other chronic health disorders.

Epilepsy in context

Part of the burden of epilepsy has to do with how it was regarded in the past. For many centuries, people with epilepsy, like people with disability, were considered as 'other' – at worst, objects on which to project society's 'shadow' or the darker side of life, including fear, negativity and prejudice. Demonic possession was (and in some cultures still is) believed to be the cause of epilepsy, and sufferers were often shunned not just by the general public but also by the medical profession. It is hardly surprising if people were forced into abnormal patterns of behaviour, which were all too easily interpreted as proof of mental abnormality.

Nineteenth-century physicians classified epilepsy as a neurosis and introduced the idea that epilepsy could take forms other than just seizures – so called 'masked epilepsy', which could show itself in all sorts of odd behaviours. Epileptic insanity formed one of three major categories of insanity as late as 1923. It is only in the twentieth century that epilepsy has become the province of the neurologist rather than the psychiatrist – it is easy to see why epilepsy and mental illness have often been confused.

The late nineteenth-century view assumed that people with epilepsy would 'degenerate', on an inevitable downward path, showing symptoms such as personality change and general deterioration. The 'epileptic personality' was believed to have certain set characteristics and to be egocentric, irritable, religious and quarrelsome, traits believed to be hereditary. It is now recognized that these early observations were of people's reaction to difficult chronic illness in much less supportive social times, when epilepsy was regarded on a par with leprosy, and colonies existed for both conditions to seclude the unfortunate sufferers from the general public. The effects of being chronically institutionalized also played a part, as did the original anticonvulsants, bromides and barbiturates, which had a powerful sedative effect, so that even when seizures were controlled, people remained too mentally numbed to function properly.

Even with the arrival of modern anticonvulsants, which controlled seizures with far less disabling effects, the prejudice against people with epilepsy remained strong and persistent, and was reflected in laws governing issues like marriage, employment and driving. To this day, in some countries in the world, it is illegal for people with epilepsy to marry. Such legislation is rooted in ancient views of epilepsy – in this case, that it is always inherited.

The epilepsy movement has done a great deal to shift these outdated prejudices. It has focused on normality and independence for those with epilepsy, and has aimed to create a positive, upbeat identity to combat stigma and ignorance. However, necessary as this may have been to redress the balance of the past, it doesn't answer all questions. For example, some people feel that, by downplaying risks, progress is held up when it comes to investigating conditions such as sudden death in epilepsy (SUDEP, covered in Chapter 1). One of the key tenets of the epilepsy movement is that epilepsy is not an illness. Yet, the medicalization of epilepsy this century has given it more dignity and helped remove it from stigma and ignorance. Epilepsy itself is not usually considered to be a disease in the usual sense of the word, but a sign of some underlying disorder characterized by a recurring disturbance in the electrical activity of the brain. The epilepsy movement and epilepsy support groups have worked hard to establish the status of epilepsy as a 'disorder' in order to raise its public image, and to dispel connotations of sickness and, in particular, contagion. (That epilepsy is contagious is one of the oldest myths there is about the condition, and does still lurk in the public consciousness.)

While current emphasis is – rightly – on the fact that people with epilepsy are just like anyone else, this may not always address issues of impairment or of just 'feeling different'. This can leave some people with epilepsy feeling frustrated or left out – such as those with difficult-to-control epilepsy, and/or other disabilities – though this does not always depend on the severity of the epilepsy or whether other difficulties are involved. In fact, some research has shown that people whose epilepsy is better controlled tend to have more anxiety, perhaps because they have more 'normality' to lose in the event of a seizure.

Being realistic does not have to mean being negative, but there is a feeling that, if the more optimistic outlook were needed historically, it is time to redress the balance and acknowledge that, while many people with epilepsy just get on with their lives, some do still often 'feel different'. The next section looks at reasons why this may be so.

Mood and behaviour

In the same way as other negative aspects of epilepsy may have been played down by the mainstream epilepsy movement, there has been outright denial of the 'epileptic personality'. While this is a hopelessly over-simplified concept, many doctors believe that certain people with epilepsy do have mood disorders which are not concerned with emotional reactions such as grief on diagnosis, but moods which exist by themselves, and which relate to electrical changes in the brain. For example, Norman Geschwind, who gave his name to the Geschwind Syndrome, studied those with 'temporal lobe seizure disorder', and found characteristic personality traits including preoccupation with philosophical or religious issues; longwindedness; altered (almost always lowered) sexuality; and irritability. Needless to say, his findings were hotly disputed by his medical colleagues, though Geschwind believed firmly in the syndrome. Another neuropsychiatrist who has done a great deal of work in this area is Dietrich Blumer, who has focused on changing moods and psychoses as part of this phenomenon. According to Blumer, mood changes are the most important mental disorders related to epilepsy and cannot be seen merely as reactions to having a difficult life situation.

So, is there any truth in all this, or is it just neurological fancy of the highest order?

Cognitive, behavioural and emotional symptoms can occur as a result of different brain disorders. In people with epilepsy, changes in thinking, personality and mood can be because of several factors.

First, the psychological aspect of epilepsy definitely has to be taken into account when considering people's experience of epilepsy. One common factor in 'moodiness' is the stress associated with adjusting to a chronic medical problem and all its implications (see the section 'Having epilepsy' below).

Mood changes may also be due to underlying brain abnormality which causes changes in electrical brain activity including seizures. This may happen as the prodrome, or build up to a seizure, described in Chapter 2, and the person with epilepsy may not necessarily be aware of his or her 'moodiness'.

> Friends and family do say I am 'moody' though I'm not always conscious of it. My husband has told me I'm particularly hard to live with in the two or three days before a seizure – in fact, I now ask him to tell me as soon as I start to 'go' because this means I can sometimes take action and stop a seizure happening, for example by lying down and taking a nap.
> *Julie*

More light may be thrown on this as medical investigative techniques advance. At some research centres, studies using advanced brain-imaging techniques are examining relationships between different behavioural symptoms and brain dysfunction in epilepsy patients. Indeed, epilepsy may well turn out to be *the* disorder of the twenty-first century, as these investigative techniques become delicate and precise enough to highlight the subtle structure and workings of the brain.

Seizure activity itself can sometimes affect feelings and outlook at depth, especially in temporal lobe epilepsy involving an aura, for example. The limbic system is closely associated with emotional life, and, when it is disturbed as in an aura, the person is likely to experience various strong emotional experiences such as fear, déjà vu, depersonalization (i.e., feeling 'not there' or detached from the scene). Over time, and especially if they began in childhood, these passing but powerful and repeated abnormal experiences, which at the time seem too real to be hallucinations, become integrated into the psychic life of the person.

Temporal lobe epilepsy itself has attracted a certain amount of attention as representing the 'sexier' end of epilepsy, and it has been linked with creativity and visionary experiences. Every artist with a claim to TLE has been drawn in, Van Gogh being one of the most typical examples! Certainly, those who experience striking hallucinations as part of an aura may resent having them dumbed down by medication.

118

For many years, I would experience visions of quite transcendant peace and love. These varied but often involved a vast white light and a vision of the two halves of the universe slowly coming together, at which point I knew that the great secret of life itself would be revealed. I also used to 'see' delightful pictures, such as parties of people in old-fashioned fancy dress, laughing and chatting. Then, hey presto! I was told I was sick, put on medication, and the visions vanished for good.

George

Seizure control is usually viewed as the criterion for success in epilepsy treatment, but some disagree!

Interestingly on this point, there are a few people, usually with lesions in the temporal lobe, who suffer psychotic illness with symptoms similar to those of paranoid schizophrenia. In this small group, the psychosis lessens when a person has more seizures, but becomes worse as the seizures are got under control – a phenomenon known as 'forced normalization'. A change in drugs can sometimes change personality 'problems'.

However, it is much more common that difficult personality traits improve when seizure frequency is reduced by the right medication. Anti-epileptic drugs are another factor which can cause changes in mood and behaviour, especially if the dose is too high, when intoxication may result, or too low, when 'breakthrough' seizures may happen.

I worked in the civil service for nine years but I believe I was pretty difficult to work with due to my trying to come to terms with epilepsy and mood swings caused by the effects of drugs. I received little support from the hospital or my parents, though my husband was wonderful and very supportive. I felt that my constant fight to cope with constant tiredness, mood swings, my feelings, my family and my drugs left my quality of life poor. The hospital more or less gave me the impression that I only had a mild form of epilepsy and should go away, stop moaning and be grateful. I stuck to my guns and 18 months ago was put on one of the new drugs. The change was amazing. My side effects vanished, I need far less sleep and honestly don't remember feeling so well. Now I am the proud owner of a provisional driving licence, something I tried not to ever think about as I knew it would probably never happen.

Lorraine

Depression

Some people with epilepsy do have a greater tendency towards depression, which can easily be understood as a natural reaction to a difficult life situation. It would not be appropriate to call this kind of psychological reaction an illness, as anyone might feel the same given the particular circumstances.

However, some neurologists believe that, as well as this kind of 'reactive depression', some people with epilepsy may be more prone to 'endogenous depression', which may need drug treatment. This type of depression is thought by some doctors to be characterized by its sudden quality – that is, it tends to come suddenly and go suddenly.

Depression is potentially serious in people with epilepsy because of the risk of suicide, which is generally estimated to be around five times higher than that of the population in general. Although this is an unpleasant statistic, it is worth mentioning because medication can be so effective in treating depression, especially if started early in the depression. It may be a matter of adjusting the dosage or type of your anti-epileptic drugs, combined if necessary with small amounts of antidepressants – a mixture which has turned life around for many former sufferers.

'Having epilepsy' – coming to terms with diagnosis

Coming to terms with epilepsy is similar to coming to terms with any other shocking major life event. There are a number of emotional responses to be gone through in the normal process of acceptance. Even if your epilepsy was diagnosed way back in childhood, you may still need to go through a grieving process in adulthood as you come to terms with the implications of epilepsy. Grief over diagnosis is very natural – in fact, it would probably be worrying if you did not grieve, as grief, including fear, anger and depression, is a necessary route to acceptance.

When told she had epilepsy, Janice went through a period of sadness which lasted several months. She felt she had lost a part of herself, or that she had lost her youth, and would look back to the days 'when I didn't have epilepsy'. She was frightened and overwhelmed by the prospect of regular doctors' appointments, medication and the general disruption into her work and family life. She was afraid of the side effects of medication, afraid of having more seizures, and afraid of dying. It took her several months to realize that in fact very little had changed, and that, as her epilepsy was swiftly controlled, she was essentially leading the same life as before. Epilepsy was in fact only a part of her life; she was still Janice.

Fear is a normal response to hearing that you have epilepsy. This fear, which underlies much of the remaining public stigma around epilepsy, is largely fear of the unknown; hence the importance already mentioned of gaining as much information as possible about your condition on diagnosis, and about epilepsy in general. You may also need support from friends, family doctor, psychiatrist and support group.

Fear of losing control, a challenge to anyone, is one of the main anxieties of epilepsy. A diagnosis of epilepsy may also bring out the fear of death. This may hardly be likely or rational, but has to do with seizures that may make you feel very vulnerable. Fear of embarrassment or of appearing different may also be even stronger than fear of death for some!

People cope with grief in different ways. Some need a lot of time alone in which to cry, to feel sad, and to think. Sometimes, being aware of and letting out these emotions may seem as if you're being weak and not coming to terms with epilepsy at all. But, being in touch with and expressing these emotions is a necessary and healthy part of grieving – better than suppressing them.

Men may generally need more help in dealing with grief, in realizing that there are coping mechanisms such as talking to others, especially those in the same situation, perhaps via an epilepsy organization. Acknowledging and dealing with these feelings is important because it will help you eventually put them behind you and move on to a more positive and productive stance.

Depression is also a natural reaction to diagnosis, though it needs to be distinguished from long-term, ongoing depression, which is dealt with separately above. Depression is a natural reaction to the burden of having seizures and their brutal interruptions into everyday life, especially if you have to lay your normal activities to one side for several hours afterwards in order to recover.

Anger is another stage. You may be angry at yourself or at life events which you feel were responsible for your epilepsy, such as a car accident – angry perhaps at your parents for passing on a 'defective gene' or for drinking or smoking during pregnancy. Anger at the medical system is another common reaction, especially given the time often involved in diagnosis, and you may need to find ways of talking to your medical carers, as this is likely to be a long-term relationship. (See Communicating with your doctor in Chapter 10.)

You may also need to come to terms with how epilepsy may affect relationships with others, as well as the best way to solve the problem of how much to tell and how much to reveal.

Acceptance takes time and has many different stages and depends partly on how good your self-acceptance and esteem were beforehand. Essentially it means accepting yourself as a normal person who happens to have seizures.

Living with uncertainty

Will I have a seizure today? Where might it take place? Can I safely go shopping on Saturday or will 'it' strike? The uncertainty factor characterizes epilepsy – not knowing exactly where and when the next seizure will strike, and what the consequences will be.

It is hard to keep positive in the face of constant uncertainty – most people need structure if they are to function well. This applies not just to the day-to-day possibility of having a seizure, but also to the larger, long-term outlook of how bad and how persistent your epilepsy will be, whether it will ever get better, and if so, when. The shadow of 'epilepsy for life' forms a major part of this, so it is important to remember that epilepsy can often get better.

A workable framework for dealing with the uncertainty of epilepsy is essential to allow you to get on with your life, make plans and maintain an optimistic, positive approach, which is fundamental to self-esteem. This may take time, and you may well need support from family and friends, doctors, nurses and perhaps epilepsy support groups. Apart from anything else, it can take several months, sometimes years, before you hit on the right medication to control your seizures, whether that's a matter of dose or the type of drug or drugs. Control can also be stop-and-start experience for some people, who have the frustrating experience of finally gaining control, only to find that a few months later seizures start again and their whole medication has to be reviewed and restarted again.

One way of dealing with uncertainty is to focus on the low probability of another seizure, and to get on with life as if it were not going to happen – or at least not today. The chances are you might well be right. Many people with epilepsy have only two, or three, or four seizures in their lifetime.

A second way is to recognize the possibility that a seizure may occur and to accept it. This involves the realization that the medical risks of a recurrent seizure are minimal and that, as has happened before, you will recover from the seizure to resume normal activity. You may even be able to accept the social consequences – people find their own way of doing this. 'I'd like to think that by having seizures, I've been able to educate the public,' says Janice.

If you do have a seizure in the face of all your positive thinking, you and your doctor can explore reasons such as forgetting medication, or not getting enough sleep. There may well be a good reason for the seizure which is in your control.

Dealing with overprotection

My mum has countless times helped me back to bed after undignified seizures and nightmares, leading to terrifying, panicking, jerking awakenings in a bed damp with sweat and urine, making me feel like an infant rather than a teenager. My seizures are now very well controlled most of the time, but in those days gone by I don't know what I would have done without my mother to comfort and reassure me, to sit at my bedside reassuring me it was safe to sleep.
Kathryn, 22

How much people with epilepsy need support is shown by Kathryn's words. It is easy to see how hard it can sometimes be to lead an independent life, and how easy to slide into dependence. This can sometimes be a fine balance. Sensible protection and support at the time of a seizure are one thing; putting a blanket restriction on all activities 'just in case', quite another – though common. Overprotection is a major issue for people with epilepsy, both by others and sometimes by themselves. It is all too natural for your nearest and dearest to want to shield you from injury of any kind, whether that's during seizures, or stupid or ignorant reactions from others. Yet, people with epilepsy, like people anywhere, need emotional freedom and independence in order to live life to the full.

Overprotection in others can be made worse by their own feelings of guilt and anxiety and may have more to do with them than you. It may not even be related to the severity of the epilepsy – often, other people's attitudes are much more of a disability than the epilepsy itself.

Janice's husband hated her going out alone shopping even though she had at most six seizures a year. Julie's partner never minded coming out to pick her up in the car after yet another seizure in a public place – it happened so often, it was just part of his life.

Epilepsy can sometimes be a hook on which to hang other anxieties and jealousies in a relationship, or may be used as a weapon with which to control those who have it. (Some people with epilepsy may also use their epilepsy as a weapon themselves, using the epilepsy to manipulate others in order to get their own way, or as a protective shield between themselves and the outside world.)

Dealing with other people's anxiety is certainly not easy. But, overprotection does need to be staved off if you are not to find yourself in relationships where you collude with people who may be only too keen to give you a dependent role. Only you can decide how much personal freedom you require, and take steps to get it.

There are various ways you can stave off overprotection. It helps to be well informed about epilepsy in general, and about your condition in particular. This includes a realistic assessment of your individual risks. How much does your epilepsy really increase the risks we all face? This information can be passed on to those close to you so that they gain an accurate estimate of the realities and risks of your particular position.

If others don't seem to take in or accept what you are saying, you may need to work harder to change the dynamic of relationships in which you are the overprotected person. You may need to learn how to say no, and how to communicate what you want without being defensive, whether you're addressing a partner, parents or other family or friends. It may also involve planning, perhaps along the following lines.

- **Stating what you want clearly.** You may have realized that there is a problem, but others may not. It is worth taking some time to plan what you are going to say. This could break down into three parts – how things are, how they affect you, and what you want to change. For example: 'I find I am staying in all the time because you're afraid of what might happen if I go out alone, and it's making me really depressed. I would like to go out to the cinema once a week.'

  This brings up another point – being specific about what you want. 'More freedom', though it is what you want, is vague. A night out a week is much more graspable. (You can always demand seven nights out a week at a later stage!)

- **Standing your ground.** Other people may agree to what you want if only out of surprise, and then come up with objections a few weeks later. For example: 'You can't go out tomorrow because I will worry too much.' This time the aim is for you to stick to what you want on the grounds that this is a reasonable request. Straight talking is often more effective here. For example: 'I want to go out on my own tomorrow.'

- **Taking action.** This is when you stop trying to communicate with words and do it with actions, such as walking out through the front door and down the road to the cinema alone.

It may take time to get your point across. Sometimes, though, it is surprising how quickly others back down and give you your space once you make up your mind what you want.

Convincing yourself

Sometimes, the overprotective person who has to be tackled is yourself, especially if you have been surrounded by too much care from childhood onwards. Inwardly you may know and admit that the life you are living is too safe, but may find it difficult to move on, and the more time passes, the more difficult it may become.

Chris, with controlled epilepsy, had married young and had stuck to a low-status, undemanding job far below his capabilities and education for ten years. His wife, a nurse, was quite happy with a relationship in which she looked after Chris in sickness and in health, and controlled his activities to the point of coming down to the job centre with him and choosing his job. But the boat was rocked when Chris met another woman in his early thirties. In contrast to Chris's wife, this woman didn't care at all about his epilepsy and was not prepared to mother him. At the same time he was offered another job with retraining which would give him important new qualifications and open up his career prospects far beyond his current status. Jolted out of his over-settled lifestyle, and very excited at the prospect of change, Chris faced a dilemma but the force of habit made it hard for him to confront it straight on. In the end, he let matters slide both with his new friend and the job offer, and Chris's rather tame but contented life went on much as before.

Of course, this kind of thing may happen to anyone, but may have more relevance for someone with epilepsy if he or she is in an overprotective relationship. Chris's story also makes the point that breaking free is not for everyone, and that some people are aware of their limits, and what lifestyle suits them.

Another reaction can be to over-compensate. A few people enter a pattern of reckless behaviour which involves not taking prescribed drugs, driving illegally and drinking heavily. This may sometimes be a part of coming to terms with epilepsy, though a part which can have heavy costs both to the person and to others around.

If overprotection is fretting you, then sooner or later you may have to take action. Getting what you really want in life requires courage and planning for everyone. Sometimes, like the rest of us, you may not even really know what you want! However, there are a number of techniques you can use to help clear your mind and let your true wishes surface.

- **Thinking back.** Think back to your earliest childhood memories. How did you view the world then? What did you enjoy? Was there anything special you wanted? Allow 20 minutes and write down what you remember, whether that's specific memories or just vague feelings associated with the time.

  You can also apply this technique to early adolescence. What were your aims? What did you hope to be? How did you envisage living your life? Again, write down the answers.

- **Asking yourself what you want.** This sounds simple but actually involves a process. Allow 30 minutes or more if you need it. One suggested technique is to visualize your awareness as a ball of white light in your mind, and then slowly take it down to your heart to see what it illuminates of what you most desire. Even if you don't get immediate insight, you may get an answer some hours or even days later.

- **Planning your ideal life.** What would you do if you could do anything you wanted? What work would you really like to be doing? What type of lifestyle or partner? Which aims would you most want to achieve? This may sound like an entry into fantasy land, and probably many people would put money and freedom as starters to the list. Put these down by all means, but the idea is to be as bold and creative as possible in all areas of your lifestyle. You may be surprised at what emerges!

Unfortunately it's beyond the scope of this book to explore these techniques further, but the Further reading section has suggestions for where to find out more, such as *Reinvent Your Life* by Jacqueline James.

Sexuality

Because my seizures are nocturnal, the prospect of sharing my bed with a man always seems to carry extra baggage. I know the sight of me convulsing and foaming at the mouth has unsettled friends I have shared a room with, and it seems a bit of a cruel thing to put a potential boyfriend through. Also, the gum guard I wear to try and stop me biting my tongue doesn't really have the same sexy connotations as various other paraphernalia! However, I've never really had any negative reactions from men or women when they've learnt about my epilepsy; usually people are just curious. One particular guy at university, while trying to convince me to sleep with him, said 'Why not – is it because you'll have a fit?' Pretty awful sex he was planning if I was going to be unconscious enough to enable a seizure!
Kathryn

The fear of what might happen during intercourse is one of the commonest reasons for men and women to feel sexually inhibited. Letting go can have connotations of extreme vulnerability for some people with epilepsy. The fear of having a seizure during lovemaking may be particularly strong among people whose seizures are sometimes triggered by hyperventilation or physical exertion; and also among those who maybe haven't yet built up a long period of sexual trust with a loving, established partner. Lack of opportunities for socializing, imposed by overprotection, may contribute to lack of sexual confidence. Fear of sex may also affect a very small percentage of people who experience sexual feelings as part of a seizure.

However, as with so many aspects of epilepsy, it seems that the fear is often worse than the reality, as seizures during sex actually happen to few people, possibly because of the well-documented fact that people enjoyably occupied tend to have fewer seizures!

There are all sorts of interesting old medical papers detailing the supposed sex lives of certain individuals with epilepsy – the man who had a safety-pin fetish, the man who could only make love mechanically in case he triggered a seizure. However, in fact, not that much research has been done in this area, and the older case histories, vivid though they are, really amount to medical curiosities. Some more modern studies report a higher incidence of sexual dissatisfaction and lack of arousal, especially among women. In one study, one third of women described themselves as dissatisfied with their overall sexual function, contrasted with 8 per cent of other women. But, a recent study of the general population by National Relate showed that 39 per cent of all women complain of loss of interest, compared with 7 per cent of men(!). This represents, for women, an increase of 50 per cent on previous estimates, and it is thought that women are no longer prepared to put up with sexual dissatisfaction as their mothers and grandmothers may have done.

In fact, most people with epilepsy should be able to have sex lives that are as 'normal' as anyone else's, with the same psychological and emotional concerns which can cause such a variety in desire and performance.

Some people are concerned about whether epilepsy drugs cause impotence. This is a possibility, especially if you notice a drop in libido soon after starting to take a certain drug. Changes in the hormones in charge of sexual behaviour also happen in epilepsy because of anti-epileptic drugs. Anti-epileptic drugs can rarely have direct effects on the areas of the brain which control sexuality and may have secondary effects on the reproductive hormones which also influence sexuality.

Occasionally repeated seizures can reduce sex drive, and, for some people with epilepsy, physiological mechanisms may play more of a part than psychological or emotional ones. Sometimes, scars or lesions in the brain may disrupt the cortical areas which control sexual desire and arousal. Several studies suggest that problems in the limbic areas of the brain especially can make sexual dysfunction more likely, and that it may be more common in individuals whose epilepsy starts from a particular region, especially the amygdala and hippocampus. It is also possible that seizures sometimes result in alterations to neurotransmitters which also result in lowered sex drive.

If impotence does occur, it is very important to discuss it with your doctor. A change of medication may make a difference – sometimes, people react to one drug with low libido, but feel better on another. Your doctor may also try adjusting medication to improve seizure control, either with your current anti-epileptic drug or drugs, or with a change of medication. Impotence should always be investigated anyway, as it can be the first sign of an underlying condition such as diabetes or heart trouble, and prompt treatment can be very effective. Other medical problems and disabilities can also affect sex life in which case advice is available from your doctor or from self-help organizations.

10

Towards empowerment

The issue of empowerment is particularly topical today, forming an important trend in epilepsy thinking and treatment. According to epilepsy organizations and the World Health Organization (WHO), as well as those with epilepsy themselves, there seems to be a general feeling that it is high time that people with epilepsy took a more active role in their treatment. 'Out of the Shadows', the health campaign launched by the WHO, is aimed at improving treatment and awareness of epilepsy, and who is better qualified to do this than those with epilepsy themselves?

Epilepsy may be different from other conditions in that the concept of taking control has far-reaching implications for those with the condition. Becoming informed about epilepsy, improving communication with your medical carers, and generally taking more responsibility for your own epilepsy and wellbeing, are all today seen as of increasing importance in coming to grips with epilepsy.

Knowing about epilepsy seems to be a key starting-point. Many studies highlight the importance of being given adequate information at the time of diagnosis and at any crisis points, such as changing drugs for pregnancy. In a condition characterized by its unpredictability, information is key in giving people a sense of control over their epilepsy.

But, many people report not receiving or having access to adequate information with regard to possible causes of their epilepsy, lifestyle implications, medication and support systems. Not being given enough information tends to make people feel more limited by epilepsy and more like victims of prejudice. Women in particular and their carers do not feel they are getting enough information and advice about issues which will have a great impact on their lives, according to the British Epilepsy Association. But, knowing about epilepsy by itself is not enough – as already stated, epilepsy varies widely. People also need to know more about their own particular form of epilepsy. In one study, patients were found to know more about epilepsy in general than about their own condition and drug regimes.

Some recent research, presented at a European Epilepsy and Society Conference, in conjunction with the International Bureau of Epilepsy, highlights certain key points as being essential to empowerment, including:

- being able to identify which factors may make seizures more likely;
- being able to explain epilepsy to others;
- understanding the importance of compliance.

The next few sections look at ways to apply these points in practice.

Identifying which factors make seizures more likely

This has to be up to the individual as everyone's epilepsy is different, though you may find it helpful to look at the list of seizure triggers in Chapter 2. Keeping a good, detailed seizure diary for at least three months is something many people find helpful, especially as it is a way of taking more responsibility for their condition. You could include:

- time of the seizure;
- what you were doing;
- anything you had to eat or drink in the preceding 24 hours;
- who you were with, and details of any social life in the day or two beforehand;
- details of your bedtime and sleep routine;
- any exercise;
- if you are a woman, any details with regard to ovulation or menstruation;
- your feelings.

Some people have been able to identify precise triggers, from lack of sleep and stressful confrontations, to certain medicines like cough mixture. You may also get a clearer idea of what kind of lifestyle suits you best, and how much stimulus. A diary is also useful as a way of monitoring the effects of anti-epileptic drugs, especially if your dose is changed, or you start taking a different drug. Some people also have typical pre-seizure moods (see prodrome, Chapter 2) and a diary may also help you be more aware of these warning signs.

Not everyone does find a link between external events and seizures, though sometimes asking a partner, close friend or your doctor to help you go over your diary may help you spot a clue you missed. However, for some, there doesn't seem to be any apparent link between outside factors and seizures.

Being able to explain epilepsy to others

Having epilepsy accentuates the normal condition of what type of persona or mask you present to the outside world, how much to tell, how much to reveal. Most people, though, will need to find some workable way of explaining epilepsy to others – friends, fellow workers, bosses, and so on. Many people evolve an explanation which suits them and produce it more or less unchanged for each new listener.

> My friends know I have epilepsy and seem to accept it. They have been interested and supportive, as are my family though the older generation seem to find it difficult to talk about disabilities including epilepsy. To them, and to new people, I explain that epilepsy is one possible reaction to tiredness or stress, just like migraine or asthma might be for others.
> *Anthea*

There are times when you might want to add more detail. One is at work, covered in Chapter 8. Another common concern is how much to tell people of the opposite sex when forming a new relationship. People may naturally feel that they want to be known first as a person, and then as a person with epilepsy, but, if epilepsy is not talked about openly from the beginning, it can become increasingly difficult to mention it. The potential risk here is of course sudden revelation by a seizure. On balance, it may be best to mention some of the basic facts so that others are prepared if a seizure does happen. True friends will appreciate the confidence shown in them by this revelation.

Understanding the importance of compliance

Compliance means taking drugs as prescribed, and is one of the most important factors in empowering people. However much they may be disliked, drugs remain the one factor which give people most control over epileptic seizures on a day-to-day basis.

Medication represents a love–hate affair for many with epilepsy – they're utterly dependent on these drugs, yet may resent having to take them in order to have a life.

> It seems so strange that those pills in a packet are the tiny points holding me on to normality – the smallest bridge to 'normal living'.
> *Anthea*

Apart from having side effects, long-term medication also involves psychological reactions which can bite deep into the psyche, becoming part of the person, especially if he or she started anti-epileptic drugs in childhood. Many people with epilepsy depend entirely on their medication in order to live a normal life; and, many people just get on with life without thinking about it too much. For some, though, having to take medication may raise all sorts of uncomfortable feelings such as feeling dependent on drugs, or a 'junkie'. Anti-epileptic drugs are a constant reminder of 'having epilepsy' and for some may dredge up reminders of the 'stigma' of the condition. Some people may not really see the point of medication or may feel over-medicated, especially if they have only had a couple of seizures. In this case it may be important to talk it over with your doctor, to help understanding of particular drugs, or to clarify why they have been prescribed, or to question whether they are indeed really needed.

Side effects, as already mentioned in Chapter 3, form a major problem for some people. Some people say they would rather have a seizure every so often than feel constantly drowsy and 'out of it'. The cosmetic effects may be unacceptable to some, too – how many young women want to take pills which they know will leave them overweight and with excess body hair?

Other reasons for non-compliance may be more pragmatic. Some people want to drink and fear their drugs will interact with alcohol. Others may simply forget, with the best of intentions, or because of unconscious or half-conscious rebellion.

Some people never forget, though. For these, drug treatment has a positive effect because it reduces worry and enables people to feel secure, independent and able to go about their activities with minimal anxiety about having a seizure – something which many with less well controlled epilepsy might envy them.

Memory

If you do forget your medication, you are not alone – poor memory is a real problem for many people with epilepsy, and can erode confidence, though they may be more aware of memory limitations through having to take medication every day – perhaps most people would find it hard to remember to do this day in, day out.

Memory can be helped along with various strategies such as wall-charts, lists, diaries (tiny computer diaries can be very helpful), and pill reminders which come in various forms, some with built-in alarms which sound at the time to take medication. Some of these strategies can help with general reminders, too.

Some people find it helpful to be more conscious of time management – planning your time may help you avoid potential stress building up if you otherwise tend to take on too much, or to respond to every call on your time.

Communicating with your doctor

Communicating better with medical professionals is a vexed question for many with epilepsy, where a typical worst scenario is having to wait several months for a hurried five-minute appointment which leaves you with a thudding heart and muscles tense in utter frustration, and in a prime condition to have another seizure!

> When I was around 17 or 18 a young up-and-coming doctor told my parents, 'Your daughter is conning you; she doesn't have epileptic seizures – she is only acting.' He told my mother to take me off phenobarbitone straight away; we knew nothing about the fact that you have to be taken off anti-epileptic drugs slowly. Next morning I felt quite ill. The last thing I remember is lying down on the sofa to go to sleep. I woke up to find myself in hospital very sick indeed, after a prolonged seizure, status epilepticus. From that day onwards, I swore that no doctor would ever do this to me again, that I would make the decisions and would also ask many questions. I learned all I could about epilepsy and if I thought the doctors were going the wrong way I would tell them.
> *Bronwen*

Yet, you and your doctors are vital partners together in dealing with your epilepsy, without which you would not have met. To summarize what has already been stated elsewhere in this book, it may help you maintain trust in your doctor if you understand the following.

- Diagnosis takes time. Many doctors prefer to monitor the situation for a while before closing in with a diagnosis of epilepsy which has such tremendous potential impact on people's lives.
- Treatment may require trial-and-error runs of medication, unlike, for example, with antibiotics, where you may be used to taking a standard dosage.
- Drugs can involve side effects – this doesn't mean they have been a failure, maybe just that they need adjusting or fine-tuning.

- Drug treatment for epilepsy does not have to last for life – there may come a time when it's appropriate to discuss the risks and benefits of withdrawal with your doctor.
- One particular situation when this should happen is before pregnancy, when your doctor should help you plan the best possible treatment for the best possible outcome.

Much research indicates that people want psychological as well as clinical advice about epilepsy from their doctors, but in practice both are often lacking. Given that most doctors are rushed off their feet, how can communication be improved?

- It is important to prepare for a doctor's appointment. It is easy to be intimidated into forgetting what you want to ask by the clinic situation, or to ask minor questions around what you really want to know, such as 'Can I drink water with my tablets?' instead of 'What is the likelihood of my seizures ever remitting?' Preparing a list of questions and concerns beforehand helps make the most of the time available.
- If you don't understand what the doctor has said, say so. You need all the information you can get about your epilepsy because it affects so many areas of life.
- Ask if it is possible to have access to a specialist epilepsy nurse who may have more time to answer many of your questions.
- If your GP or neurologist cannot answer your questions to your satisfaction, seek a specialist opinion (not all neurologists specialize in epilepsy), perhaps with the help and advice of an epilepsy organization.

Tackling stigma

In a recent BEA survey, 97 per cent of respondents still felt stigma to be an issue for people living with epilepsy. While the role of epilepsy associations in educating the public is important, perhaps the best advocate for epilepsy is the person with epilepsy. Usually, just information is what is needed to embarrass others into retracting casually held prejudices and half-ideas about epilepsy.

> Ignorance is the main problem, not prejudice. People don't want to be with you in case you have a seizure, and they would be frightened, not knowing what to do and how to react. Certainly, you soon find out who really cares when you're lying flat on the ground!
> *Bronwen*

The fight against stigma is an ancient one, dating back to a time when medicine was closely linked with religion and diseases were believed to be visitations from demons or gods. Hippocrates, born in 406 BC, led the fight against ignorance and stigma on the so-called Sacred Disease, saying it was no more sacred than any other disease. 'Men ought to know that from nothing else but the brain comes joys, delights, laughter, sorrows, griefs, despondency and lamentations . . . And by the same organ we become mad and delirious, and fears and terrors assail us.'

With the increasingly sophisticated medicalization of epilepsy, perhaps the twenty-first century will at last see these words being accepted and believed.

Again, being informed about epilepsy will help you deal with other people's beliefs about epilepsy, whether openly stated or not. Uninformed or unthinking comments, though likely to set your blood boiling, may actually be easier to answer than unstated beliefs which nevertheless influence other people's attitudes and actions towards you. Of course, it is not your job to set the world right about epilepsy, but you can influence those around you, and how active you want to be depends on you and your individual style. This could vary widely, from providing information leaflets from one of the epilepsy organizations, to going back to a shop where you have had a seizure to explain facts about epilepsy to those who witnessed it, to just getting on with your life so that you are known first and foremost as a person who just happens to have epilepsy.

One point, which perhaps doesn't go as far back as Hippocrates but is old enough, is how much stigma is real, and how much it is perceived. It can sometimes be easy to imagine negative responses where none exist, especially if your self-esteem is not great. Certainly, good self-confidence is key in tackling fear of what others may think. Lack of confidence can erode quality of life, and impact on wellbeing, lifestyle and health. Sometimes, coming to terms with your own fears about epilepsy may need to be tackled before you can change other people's attitudes.

Boosting confidence

This can take time and be an ongoing process, as it can tend to slip temporarily if you are tired or under the weather. 'Having epilepsy', poor memory and concentration, slow thinking, mood swings – there are many variables which may combine to affect confidence. However, confidence is key to having any control over your life, and there is a great deal you can do to maintain self-esteem.

- Have as much control as possible over your epilepsy. This means taking responsibility for your medical care, including taking medication regularly, initiating discussions with your doctor, and preparing for appointments as discussed above.
- Find out about epilepsy in general. Many studies have shown that the best-adjusted people are those who are best informed.
- Take responsibility for informing others accurately about your epilepsy, and selectively. Not everyone has to know. However, people with whom you spend a lot of time will probably appreciate your trust in them, and it may also have practical implications if ever they do have to deal with a seizure when in your company.
- Don't be afraid of speaking out for your rights as a person who happens to have epilepsy. Taking action may change things and will probably help your self-esteem.
- Try and arrange to witness a seizure. You may find it helpful to see a video which shows the particular type of seizure from which you suffer, typically the part of yourself which is invisible to you. Other medical sufferers can look in a mirror. This may help you understand and deal with others' reactions when you have one.
- Accept realistic limitations which may in reality be only slightly different from those of everyone else. How many people do you know who actually go scuba-diving?

What to do in the event of a seizure

Bronwen's words above show clearly that people may back off because they are afraid they won't know what to do if a person does have a seizure. This is natural. It can be very upsetting to witness tonic-clonic convulsive seizures, even for nurses who see them every day. However, knowing what to do in the event of a seizure is one major practical way in which fear of epilepsy can be tackled.

Attacks cannot be stopped, so do not try and restrain the person during a seizure, or let other people interfere, crowd round, or try and touch the person.

Convulsive seizures:

- Put something soft under the person's head and only move them if they're in danger (e.g., in the road).
- Do not put anything in the person's mouth.
- Once convulsions have stopped, roll the person on to his side into the recovery position.
- Wipe away any saliva and if the person is still breathing with difficulty, check there is nothing in the mouth such as food.
- Stay with the person to help reassure them until he feels able to get on with his activities, or arrange transport so he can go home and rest.

Non-convulsive seizures:

These seizures vary and may need different responses. In prolonged confusion:

- Gently guide the person away from obvious dangers such as traffic.
- Speak calmly and gently to the person to help her reorientate herself.
- Stay with the person until she is able to resume what she was doing. Bear in mind she may be confused for some time after the attack, and because of this may sound aggressive, so it may be best to stay fairly quiet until she has come round fully and is able to manage alone.

Get medical help if:

- A seizure lasts longer than five minutes and you don't know how long they usually last.
- The person has trouble breathing after a seizure.
- The person has hurt themselves badly during a seizure.

Finally . . . adjusting to epilepsy – a constant process

Adjusting to epilepsy can be an evolving process. Many people's epilepsy is dynamic, not static. Just when you've come to terms with the epilepsy you have, seizures may change their type and intensity, for example, going from being nocturnal to happening during the day. While the changes should obviously be reported to the doctor and treated accordingly, this means of course that you have to come to terms with 'having epilepsy' all over again.

Equally, though, the same process means that many people may find that their epilepsy improves as time goes on, with seizures becoming less intense, less troubling, and sometimes going away altogether. Whatever the nature of your epilepsy, it is worth taking steps to get it thoroughly reviewed at intervals.

Meanwhile, it is hoped that this book has suggested some ways in which to deal with it more effectively. As Paracelsus (1490–1541) said, love is the highest level of medicine, and you owe this kind of care to yourself, by trying to ensure you get optimal medical care, and by looking after your daily lifestyle, health and general wellbeing as much as possible.

Further reading

These are the books and references used in this book which you may find useful as further reading.

Appleton, Richard and Gibbs, John, *Epilepsy in Childhood and Adolescence*, Martin Dunitz 1995.

Appleton, Richard, Chappell, Brian and Beirne, Margaret, *Your Child's Epilepsy: A Parent's Guide*, Class Publishing 1997.

Betts, Tim and Crawford, Pamela, *Women and Epilepsy*, Martin Dunitz 1998.

Chadwick, David and Usiskin, Susan, *Living with Epilepsy*, Macdonald Optima (2nd edn) 1991.

Chappell, Brian and Crawford, Pamela, *Epilepsy at Your Fingertips*, Class Publishing 1999.

Fenwick, Peter and Fenwick, Elizabeth, *Living with Epilepsy*, Bloomsbury Publishing 1996.

Freeman, John M., Kelly, Millicent T. and Freeman, Jennifer B., *The Epilepsy Diet Treatment: An Introduction to the Ketogenic Diet*. Available from bookshops or from Demos Publications, 386 Park Avenue South, New York, New York 10016 (tel. 800–532–8663).

Freeman, John M., Vining, Eileen P. G. and Pillas, Diana J., *Seizures and Epilepsy in Childhood: A Guide for Parents*, Baltimore: Johns Hopkins University Press 1997.

Glenville, Marilyn, *Natural Alternatives to HRT*, Kyle Cathie 1997.

Goffman, Erving, *Stigma*, Englewood Cliffs NJ: Prentice-Hall, 1963.

Hanscomb, A. and Hughes, L., *Family Health Guide: Epilepsy*, Ward Lock 1995.

Hopkins, Anthony and Appleton, Richard, *Epilepsy – The Facts*, Oxford University Press (2nd edn) 1996.

James, Jacqueline, *Reinvent Your Life*, Hodder & Stoughton 1996.

James, Jacqueline, *Take Control of Your Life*, Hodder & Stoughton 1995.

Kitzinger, Sheila, *Birth over Thirty-Five*, Sheldon Press 1982.

Kitzinger, Sheila, *Pregnancy and Childbirth*, Penguin 1989.

Laidlaw, Mary and Laidlaw, John, *People with Epilepsy: How They Can Be Helped*, Churchill Livingstone 1984.

Laplante, Eve, *Seized: Temporal Lobe Epilepsy as a Medical, Historical, and Artistic Phenomenon*, HarperCollins 1994.

FURTHER READING

Lewis, David, *10-Minute Time and Stress Management*, Piatkus 1999.

Marshall, Fiona, *Coping with Postnatal Depression*, Sheldon Press 1994.

Marshall, Fiona, *Your Child, Epilepsy*, Element Books 1998.

Marshall, Fiona, *The Natural Way, Epilepsy*, Element Books 1998.

Oxley, Jolyon and Smith, Jay, *The Epilepsy Reference Book*, Faber and Faber 1991.

Sacks, Oliver, *Migraine*, Picador 1993.

Sander, L. and Thompson, P., *Epilepsy: A Practical Guide To Coping*, Crowood Press 1989.

Scrambler, Graham, *Epilepsy*, The Experience of Illness Series, Tavistock/Routledge 1989.

Schneider, Joseph W. and Conrad, Peter, *Having Epilepsy: The Experience and Control of Illness*, Philadelphia: Temple University Press, 1983.

Temkin, Oswei, *The Falling Sickness*, Baltimore: Johns Hopkins University Press, 1945.

Thomas, Caroline, *Epilepsy: A Holistic Approach*, Images Publishing 1993. Available from Nutricentre, 7 Park Crescent, London W1N 3HE.

Trimble, M. R., *Women and Epilepsy*, Wiley 1991.

Walker, M. C. and Shorvon, S., *Understanding Epilepsy*, Family Doctor Publications, in association with the British Medical Association, 1995.

Useful addresses

British Epilepsy Association
Anstey House
40 Hanover Square
Leeds LS3 1BE
Tel: 0113 243 9393
Fax: 0113 242 8804
E-mail: epilepsy@bea.org.uk
Helpline: 0800 30 90 30
Website: www.epilepsy.org.uk

Information, nationwide and local support, newsletter, leaflets and videos on several aspects of epilepsy.

National Society for Epilepsy
Chesham Lane
Chalfont St Peter
Gerrards Cross
Bucks SL9 0RJ
Tel: 01494 601300
Fax: 01494 871927
Website: http://www.erg.ion.uvl.ac/NSEhome

Information, leaflets, videos, network of community self-help groups, training and training packages for health and other professionals; residential care, respite care and assessment for adults with severe epilepsy and learning difficulties.

Other epilepsy associations
Brainwave: The Irish Epilepsy Association
249 Crumlin Road
Dublin 12
Tel: +353 1 4557500

Epilepsy and the Young Adult (EYA)
13 Crondace Road
London SW6 4BB

Epilepsy Association of Scotland
48 Govan Road
Glasgow G51 1JL
Tel: 0141 427 4911

Epilepsy Bereaved?
PO Box 1777
Bournemouth BH5 1YR

For a Better Life with Epilepsy (FABLE)
The Old Bank
239–241 Crookes
Sheffield S10 1TF
Tel/fax: 0114 268 4977
Helpline: 0800 521 629

Fetal Anti Convulsant Syndrome (FACS)
Linda Hamilton
Newton of Brux
Glenkindie
Aberdeenshire AB33 8RX
Tel: 019755 71340

Friends of Landau-Kleffner Syndrome (F.O.L.K.S.)
PO Box 749
Erith
Kent DA8 3UA
Helpline: 0870 8470707

Gamma-knife Surgery Support Organization
E-mail: gammaknife@lineone.net
Fax: 01223 863347

International Bureau for Epilepsy
PO Box 21, NL-2100 AA Heemstede
Holland
Tel: +31 23 29 10 19/23 74 11
Fax: +31 23 47 01 19
E-mail: ibe@xs40all.nl

An international organization for people with epilepsy and their friends; English spoken.

International League Against Epilepsy (ILAE)
Department of Health and Human Services
National Institute of Health
Building 31
Bethseda
Maryland 20892
USA

For doctors and other professionals.

Ketogenic diet contacts
Call the BEA Helpline for local hospitals which may consider the diet or consult your neurologist.

Mersey Region Epilepsy Association
The Glaxo Centre
Norton Street
Liverpool L3 8LR
Tel: 0151 298 2666

Support Dogs
PO Box 447
Sheffield S6 6YZ
Tel/fax: 0114 257 7997

For seizure-alert dogs. A registered charity. Each dog costs around £1,500 to train. No charge is made to the person with epilepsy and funding is from sponsorship and donations.

Wales Epilepsy Association
15 Chester Street
St Asaph
Denbighshire LL17 0RE
Tel/fax: 01755 584444
Helpline: 0345 413774

The Epilepsy Foundation of America has launched a global internet project to speed progress in genetic research, the Epilepsy Gene Discovery Project. Experts involved in the project believe that genetic factors may play far more of a part in epilepsy than is currently known, involving a large and diverse group of genes. Visit the EFA Gene Discovery Web Site at (http://www.epilepsygene.org/epi/). Confidentiality is guaranteed, and families are free to withdraw from the probject at any time.

Other useful addresses and contact numbers
Cry-sis
Tel: 020 7404 5011

Help for parents of crying babies.

DVLA (Driver and Vehicle Licensing Agency)
Drivers' Medical Unit
Longview Road
Morriston
Swansea SA99 1TU

Enquiries about driving licences.

Employment Service
National Office
Sanctuary Building
Great Smith Street
London SW1P 3BT

Footprints
Tel: 01706 819200

Helps parents communicate with health professionals.

La Leche League helpline
Tel: 020 7242 1278

Help and advice on breastfeeding.

National Childbirth Trust
Alexandra House
Oldham Terrace
London W3 6NH
Tel: 020 8992 8637

Help and advice on birth, breastfeeding and mothering; local support groups.

Rare Disorders Alliance – UK (RDA–UK)
Tel: 020 7383 3555
E-mail: rda@cafamily.org.uk

Royal College of Midwives
15 Mansfield Street
London W1M 0BE
Tel: 020 7872 5100

Royal Society for the Prevention of Accidents (RoSPA)
Edgbaston Park
353 Bristol Road
Birmingham B5 7ST
(SAE please)
Tel: 0121 248 2000

Index

INDEX

ketogenic diet 56–8

labour 85–6; pain relief during 85; seizure during 86; vomiting during 86 *see also* birth
lamotrigine 40, 65
lavender oil 53
law and employment 103
learning disability 7
Lennox, Dr William 115
Lennox-Gastaut syndrome 23
levoreticam 42
Lewis, Dr David 90
limitations, self-imposed 2
LINAC surgery 50
lobes, of brain 3, 20
luteinizing hormone (LH) 62

magnesium 96
magnetic resonance imaging *see* MRI
manganese 96
massage 53–4
Maudsley Hospital 51
medical history 30–2, 73, 74
medication *see* drugs
meditation 98–100
memory 21, 133
men 8–9, 23, 121
menopause 69
menstruation 24, 61–5, 71, 131
migraine 7–8, 28
mind control techniques 51–2
minor motor epilepsy *see* Lennox-Gastaut syndrome
misdiagnosis 27
monotherapy 38
mood changes 52, 117–19
MRI (magnetic resonance imaging) 34, 49
music therapy 100
musicogenic epilepsy 100, 105
myoclonic seizure 18

narcolepsy 29
National Relate 128
National Society for Epilepsy (NSE) 8, 80, 142
nausea during pregnancy 82–3
neuronal migration 6
nocturnal seizures 21
Non-Epileptic Attack Disorder (NEAD) 29
nuchal fold scan 83

occipital lobe 20
oestrogen 61–3
operation *see* surgery

osteoporosis 70–1
overprotection 2, 123–5, 126
ovulation 131
oxcarbazepine 42, 65

panic attacks 30
paraldehyde 38
parietal lobe 20
paroxysmal choreoathetosis 29
partial seizures 16, 19–21 *see also* simple partial seizures; complex partial seizures
penicillin 25
periods *see* menstruation
PET scan 34
petit mal see absence seizures
phenobarbitone 41, 65, 88
phenytoin 40, 65, 66, 77
photosensitivity 23, 24, 98
pill, contraceptive 62
piracetam 41, 65
polycystic ovary syndrome 68–9
positron emission tomography *see* PET scan
post-ictal automatisms 21
postnatal depression (PND) 87
posture 99
pre-conception care 73–81
pre-eclampsia 86–7
pregnancy 5, Ch 6; complications of 86–7; constipation 83; maximizing chances of 67–8; nausea 82–3; preparing for *see* pre-conception care; tests and checks 83–4; warning signs of 86–7
pre-menstrual tension 63–5
primary generalized epilepsy 5
primidone 42, 65, 66, 88
prodromata and prodrome 25–6, 52
progesterone 61–3; natural 62
prognosis 13–14
protein 94
pseudoseizures *see* Non-Epileptic Attack Disorder
psychological component of seizures 51

qualifications of alternative therapists 54
quality of life 90

reflex epilepsy 24–5
reflexology 54
relationships 114–15, 127–9
remission 12–14
responsibility, importance of taking for own health 31–2
Rett syndrome 23
Reynolds, Dr Edward 58
rosemary oil 53

149

INDEX